Utilization of Health Personnel

A Five Hospital Study

Harold M. Goldstein
Morris A. Horowitz

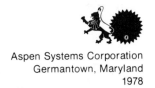

Aspen Systems Corporation
Germantown, Maryland
1978

Library of Congress Cataloging in Publication Data

Goldstein, Harold M., 1930—
Utilization of health personnel.

Bibliography: p. 151
Includes index.
1. Hospitals—Staff. 2. Hospitals—Job descriptions.
3. Allied health personnel—Employment. 4. Hospitals
—United States—Staff. 5. Allied health personnel—
Employment—United States. I. Horowitz, Morris Aaron,
joint author. II. Title. [DNLM: 1. Economics,
Hospital—United States. 2. Health manpower—Utilization—
United States. W76 G622u]
RA972.5.G64   658.3'7'36211   78-12011
ISBN   0-89443-080-7

Library of Congress Catalog Card Number: 78-12011
ISBN: 0-89443-080-7
Printed in the United States of America
1 2 3 4 5

To

Seth, Mark, and Joel

This study was funded by the Office of Research and Development Education and Training Administration, United States Department of Labor. This study does not necessarily represent the official opinion or policy of the Employment and Training Administration or Northeastern University. The authors are solely responsible for the contents of the study.

Contents

Tables

Acknowledgements

This study began in 1973 and ran concurrently with several other research projects at the Center for Medical Manpower Studies of the Department of Economics, Northeastern University. We are reporting on this study now because we have reached a point where conclusions can be drawn and recommendations made. We should note, however, that our contacts with the hospitals in this study continue, and if substantial or significant developments occur we will report on them at a later date.

We are indebted to a large number of people who gave freely of their time and ideas. To Dr. Howard Rosen, director of the Office of Research and Development, Employment and Training Administration, United States Department of Labor, we owe our greatest appreciation for his ideas, encouragement, and support. We owe special thanks to Mr. William Throckmorton, Project Monitor, and to others at the Office of Research and Development who assisted in the design and implementation of the project.

We are particularly grateful to the administrators and staff of the five hospitals who graciously allowed our research team to work for many hours in their hospitals.

Many persons at the Center for Medical Manpower Studies worked on the study. Kathy Calore was responsible for transforming the interview data into statistical tables, Nancy Benotti assisted in editing the manuscript, and Alec Cheloff helped in many ways throughout the study. Pat McCarville, Bonnie Campbell, Katharine Wilkins, Lois McLennan, Pauline Sayers, and other members of our secretarial staff worked with diligence and great patience in typing the manuscript and the many pages of statistical tables. Our sincere thanks to all of them.

We also wish to express our appreciation to William A. Frolich, Sarah Evans, and Pauline Simons for their editorial assistance.

This study does not necessarily represent the official opinion or policy of the Employment and Training Administration or of Northeastern University. The authors are solely responsible for its contents.

1

Introduction

Over the past decade the costs of health care have been rising at a faster rate than the overall rate of inflation in the nation. There are many indicators that medical care costs are likely to continue to rise sharply in the future. The consumer price index (CPI) rose 7.7 percent (not including medical services) in 1975, while the medical care services of the CPI rose 10.3 percent, hospital service charges rose 13 percent, and physicians' fees rose by 11.8 percent. In 1965 health care expenditures represented 5.9 percent of gross national product (GNP); ten years later health care expenditures had increased 41 percent to represent 8.3 percent of GNP. Through the first three months of 1976, medical care services rose at a 14 percent annual rate, physicians' fees at a 14.2 percent rate, and hospital service charges at a 20.1 percent rate. The CPI during this period rose at a rate of only 2.4 percent (not including medical services).[1]

During the last decade, especially since 1972, an implicit public policy has emerged to limit the runaway costs of medical care in the United States. The federal government has shown its interest and influence in cost containment by the recent passage of two bills, the Social Security Amendments of 1972 and the National Health Planning and Resource Development Act of 1974. In addition, other third-party payers and certificate of need

1

committees of individual states have expanded their concern and influence to the specifics of growing health care costs. The rate setting committees of individual states and consumer group organizations have also increasingly emphasized the need to justify higher hospital costs and charges.

As a result hospital administrators, chiefs of services, and boards of trustees of health providers have genererally paid more attention to the monitoring of changes in medical costs, expenditures, and charges. Overall, however, visible results of all the increased attention are perhaps difficult to observe or document. As we have already noted, over the period 1965-1975 price increases for health care services far exceeded the average increases in the CPI.

Factors in Rising Health Care Costs

An historical perspective may shed some light on the reasons for the substantial increases in hospital costs. In general, hospitals had been established as charitable institutions for the poor, and it was only after World War II that middle and upper income groups began to use their services to any extent. Many who worked in hospitals before 1940 either contributed their services or were paid a very meager wage. Since then there have been substantial increases in the wages of health personnel. However, even despite the increases, the average wage of hospital workers in 1977 lagged behind that of their counterparts in the industrial sector.

Over the last several decades there has been a very substantial increase in the utilization of sophisticated health care technology, which has resulted in increased specialization among health care workers with higher levels of formal education, increased amounts of in-service education, or on-the-job training. The increased emphasis on medicine has had varying effects. On the one hand we are participating in increasing numbers of consultations, laboratory tests, x-rays, and other such services; on the other, the American consumer is obliged the pay the burgeoning costs of these services. Other factors in the soaring costs of medical care are the general growth of the American population and the increased demand for health services—the result of higher levels of affluence and education within the consuming public. All these factors contribute to the escalation of health care costs.

Labor Costs

Labor costs are a very substantial proportion of the total costs of any hospital or other health provider. The costs of labor as a percentage of total expenses for all United States hospitals had increased from 56 percent in 1946 to a high of 66.4 percent in 1960. Since 1960, however, labor costs as a percentage of total hospital expenses have declined every year, reaching 54.2 percent in 1976.[2] It should be noted that these percentages vary with the type of hospital.

For example, in 1976 in nongovernmental, not-for-profit, short-term, general and special hospitals, payroll represented 52.3 percent of total expenses. For state and local government, short-term, general and special hospitals, payroll represented 51.8 percent of total expenses. Since these percentages generally do not include the costs of physicians' services, the figures are on the low side. Approximately 25 percent of all physicians in the United States are contractual physicians, and the remaining 75 percent all have staff privileges in anywhere from two to ten hospitals. The total wage charge for contractual physicians is a somewhat confusing issue. If a teaching hospital is involved, a major portion of the salary of the physician, intern, or resident is absorbed by the medical college, even though many teaching hospital physicians are almost totally contractual.

Management

If cost containment is indeed a goal of hospitals and other health providers, a substantial effort must be made to manage more effectively the broad range of health personnel. Health provider management and administration must make strong efforts to expand the productivity of its health care employees. One of the first issues to be faced is that of the quantity and quality of health care administrators. The daily administrative functions of running a hospital are usually in the hands of middle echelon health care administrators (MEHCAs), and without their full and enthusiastic cooperation, it would be difficult, if not impossible, to improve the productivity of health personnel.

At present the market for health administrators is extremely disorganized, and there appears to be a split in the link between the demand and the need for administrators and individuals with the proper educational credentials. In effect, the system has developed so rapidly that a disequilibrium has developed in the market. This is indicated by the lack of specific descriptions of necessary qualifications within personnel departments in hospitals and by the haphazard nature in which many positions are now filled. Occupational ladders are not clearly defined, and many positions are filled by physicians and others who are not trained for managerial functions. According to the Kellogg study, only one in four health administrators has had any formal training in the field, and the use of improperly or poorly trained individuals is a major source of upward pressure on costs in the health care system.[3]

An important factor in the current situation is that a substantial proportion of middle echelon health care administrators are probably not especially qualified or equipped to pursue major goals such as cost containment or the increased labor productivity that depends on improvements in job satisfaction, general morale, and employee relations.

Training and Utilization of Health Care Personnel

Fifty years ago the hospital often symbolized an employer of last resort. The enormous increase in the demand for hospital services and the increased complexities of medical technology have drastically altered this image in recent years. The rapid growth and increasing sophistication of health care providers are changing the nature of many hospital positions. As a result, the role of hospitals in providing health employee education and training is slowly expanding.

One must recognize that meaningful, well-paid jobs with realistic opportunities for advancement do not seem readily available in the health industry for the disadvantaged and for ethnic minorities. For various reasons health providers and professional associations of various occupations have established employment barriers. Education, training, and experience requirements, certification and licensing commonly restrict the potential supply of employees. It is difficult to avoid the conclusion that the disadvantaged are usually the first to be denied entry into jobs with advancement possibilities.

When health providers, in isolated but significant examples, have modified formal education and training requirements, there has been no measurable impact on patient care. Of course, we recognize that the validity of this observation is somewhat difficult to establish. The end product of quality medical care in most instances can be measured only by gross guidelines such as infant mortality rates, morbidity, mortality, and longevity—outcomes that are often controlled more by the consumer than by health care providers. Still, our research in the area of health personnel utilization over the last decade indicates that significant modifications can be made in the hiring-in requirements of health providers with overall positive results. If the hiring requirements can be modified successfully by some health providers, one can legitimately assume that most other health providers could make similar changes and achieve satisfactory results.

Can an individual with substantially less training than that of an MD be taught to use a sphygmomanometer (blood pressure measuring device)? Is it possible for an individual with one year of proper medical training to qualify for performing electroencephalography (that is, taking and recording—not reading—electric currents developed in the brain)? Could similar training requirements realistically be applied to electrocardiography (that is, the taking of graphic records of the electric currents emanating from the heart muscle)? The answer to all these questions is yes, though the three terms alone are probably enough to intimidate the average layman.

What we are suggesting is certainly no revolutionary notion. It is common to break down long, complicated procedures into meaningful but less complex functions. Entry-level health personnel have been trained on the job to perform the duties of electrocardiogram (EKG) and electroencephalograph (EEG) technicians. Nursing assistants, licensed practical nurses (LPNs with eighteen months of formal training), and registered nurses (RNs with three years of schooling) utilize tools such as sphygmomanometers and EKG and EEG equipment. Laboratory technicians in many private laboratories in the large cities of the United States regularly use such equipment on patients sent to them by physicians.

The occupational structure of the health care industry as it now stands does not allow significant upward mobility or even lateral mobility. Entry-level positions are generally dead-end occupations. Morale is low and the turnover rate very high, both of which lead to poor performance and potentially higher costs.

Over the last decade in the United States and elsewhere, experimental efforts have been made to restructure the occupational hierarchy of health providers and to create realistic occupational ladders. These attempts have been few in number and have had little overall impact. In the future, considerable effort and pressure by consumers, providers, and government will be required to institute change. It is our belief that meaningful work opportunities can be made available in the health care industry for the fairly large number of persons now locked out of this field, many of whom are unemployed or underemployed. In addition, many of those employed in various entry-level jobs can be offered improved work opportunities. Further, we believe change in the structure of health care providers can be accomplished without additional risk to the consuming public or a lowering of current standards of medical care.

The study that is the subject of this report was aimed at clarifying specific issues. In this study, we addressed the following questions: To what extent is there substantial overlap in the performance of medical functions by various categories of health personnel? If indeed substantial overlap is occurring, what impact does it have on health care employees with respect to the utilization of their time, their morale, turnover rates, and general job satisfaction? What specific types of efforts have promise for resolving the issues and problems discussed? What are the broad implications of changes in health care job structures on the delivery of health care and the overall utilization and employment of those persons currently excluded from the industry or artificially maintained in dead-end jobs?

In our attempt to answer these questions, we examined the medical functions of a select group of health personnel employed in five hospitals of varying characteristics. Our object was to test the general validity of the recommendations that were the product of two of our previous studies. The background material that these studies provided is the subject of chapters 2 and 3.

2

Earlier Health Personnel Studies

If the market for health care employees operated efficiently, with no artificial barriers, supply and demand interaction would ultimately correct shortages. Health providers would act to retain employees, attract new employees from other institutions, restructure hiring standards, and modernize compensation policies. In addition, proficiency examinations would receive more attention, and training programs would be explored along with new sources of recruitment.

The Labor Market

A labor market study of licensed practical nurses (LPNs) and medical technologists in Chicago and St. Louis hospitals found persistent and serious, although not critical, shortages in the mid-1960s.[1] The recruitment of health personnel by hospitals reporting shortages was limited to mild competition with area hospitals for the active available employee pool. Occupational entry routes were still narrowly prescribed in terms of training and education. Although area hospitals had accepted members of minority groups, especially LPNs, and although graduates of LPN schools in St. Louis were about the same racial mix as the hospital work force, the lengthy lists of qualified LPN applicants were nonetheless dominated by blacks. The study also found that the quality of services was lower than it would have been had sufficient numbers of qualified personnel been employed by hospitals.

In many instances, reported health employee shortages tended to reflect budgeted positions and past experience in hiring and turnover, and not necessarily the real need for qualified personnel. Under these conditions, even if skilled personnel had been available to fill listed vacancies, there was certainly no guarantee that they would have been employed. The use of medical technicians and nurse's aides as substitutes for medical technologists and registered nurses or LPNs was found to indicate either a shortage of higher-level personnel or an attempt to control costs by using lower-paid employees to perform functions traditionally reserved for higher-level personnel.

This attempt at cost containment had another result. Few adjustments in wages or market conditions took place, indicating that individual hospitals were unwilling or unable to undertake a reordering of personnel affairs. Overall, the result was a high job vacancy rate, which can be considered one criterion of a labor shortage.

During the late 1960s national data tended to confirm a persistent lag in earnings in health occupations, despite widespread reports of labor shortages. Average annual earnings in private nonagricultural industry were $4,920 in 1965, compared to $3,308 in medical and other health services.[2] A survey of hospital workers in March 1969 showed average weekly earnings in a number of health occupations remaining substantially below those for production workers in the durable goods sector. A nurse's aide at that time earned an average of $76 weekly, which represented 56 percent of the average weekly earnings of a production worker; a psychiatric aide's average weekly earnings of $96 represented 70 percent; an LPN's $99 represented 72 percent; and an x-ray technician's $120 represented 88 percent.[3]

Poor working conditions and relatively low wages have resulted in a predominantly female work force in the health care industry. The Greenfield study, based on national data for the mid-1960s, found that 80 percent of allied health workers in positions not requiring a college degree were women, many of whom entered the health field five, ten, or twenty years after leaving high school.[4] Greenfield pinpointed two other characteristics of the health industry that tended to account for the predominance of women in the work force. The study found a collection of small, quasi-independent labor markets for health personnel, each composed of separate and rigidly defined occupations. The markets for the lower-skill levels tended to be local or regional. These fragmented labor markets led to improper use of less-skilled employees in dead-end occupations, huge turnover rates, and job dissatisfaction. In addition, the study found that these relatively small health units, which were for the most part charitable, nonprofit hospitals, had little if any administrative hierarchy separate from the professional hierarchy, a condition that further limited upward mobility and male employment. The entry of more men into these occupations would tend to stabilize the work force and raise wages,[5] since relatively few men are attracted by low-paying positions that offer little prospect of advancement.

Barriers to Employment

The first pilot study in the health personnel field undertaken by the Center for Medical Manpower Studies, Northeastern University, began in 1967.[6] Entitled *Hiring Standards for Paramedical Manpower,* its purpose was to identify any artificial barriers to employment that might exist in a sample of hospitals in the Greater Boston area. In an effort to define realistic job requirements, detailed data were gathered on hiring requirements, job performance, and educational and professional backgrounds of employees in selected health occupations, as well as information on general characteristics of the occupations (for example, promotional possibilities and training on the job). The study involved twenty hospitals, including private, municipal, and veterans' units, and covered 524 employees in twenty-two health occupations. The occupations were selected to cover a broad range of technical occupations requiring a wide variety of training.

Since the Boston area contained relatively more health personnel than the typical metropolitan area in the United States, it was recognized that health personnel problems in Greater Boston may differ from those in other parts of the United States. It was also recognized that the twenty-two occupations studied may not be statistically representative of all occupations. Nevertheless, it was felt that a number of generalizations were warranted, even though each finding, conclusion, or recommendation might not have universal applicability.

Advancement Potential

The report documented high turnover and poor job prospects for health personnel. Workers were asked what occupational level they hoped to attain and how long they had been working at their current occupations. In only six of eighteen jobs did a majority of employees expect to advance beyond their current job (see table 1). In thirteen of the jobs, at least two-fifths of the employees had been in the occupation for less than three years. Three years was chosen somewhat arbitrarily as a time long enough for the employee both to display an attachment to the job and to make a fairly realistic assessment of the chances for advancement.

Actual Task Performance and Hiring Standards

The study examined the difficulty of tasks performed, the amount of time spent on tasks of *varying* difficulty, and the amount of task overlap between different occupations. A strong effort was made to compare tasks within the hierarchy of the selected health occupations. For example, higher-skilled personnel such as LPNs were juxtaposed with lower-skilled nurse's aides (NAs), histotechnologists with histotechnicians, and so forth. The pilot study did not include occupational levels above LPNs in nursing and general medical care. Respondents were asked to indicate on a list of tasks normally performed in their positions whether they performed each function and the amount of time spent on each.

Table 1. Allied Health Workers' Attitudes toward Advancement and Tenure in Present Occupation, in 20 Boston Hospitals, 1968

Occupation	Total number interviewed	Percent who believed they would not advance beyond present job	Percent working in occupation 3 years or less
Dietary aid	21	96	19
X-ray developing machine operator	9	89	22
Physical and corrective therapy aide	5	80	60
Nurse's aide	51	67	50
Microbiology technician	19	67	42
Medical records technician	9	67	22
Histology technician	12	67	33
Psychiatric aide	26	62	65
Licensed practical nurse	54	59	51
Inhalation therapist	17	53	47
Hematology technican	23	52	59
EEG technician	10	50	70
Radiation therapist	12	42	50
Blood bank technician	12	42	42
Biochemistry technician	22	41	32
EKG technician	16	38	44
X-ray technician	33	27	55
Cytotechnician	7	14	43

Source: Horowitz and Goldstein, *Hiring Standards for Paramedical Manpower*, Summarized from tables, 4, 10, 11, 19, 25, 44-49, 57-62, 81-85, 91-95, 110-112, and 118-120.

The process of developing task lists for each occupation involved the cooperation of supervisors, instructors, and experienced employees in each field. On the advice of these consultants, the tasks were ranked in order of complexity, from the easiest or most routine to the most unusual or difficult. *Easy* or *difficult* did not refer to physical exertion but to the level of formal training or experience considered necessary to accomplish the work. For example, the nursing tasks identified as easy were cleaning rooms, washing and dressing deceased persons, recording fluid intake and output, performing routine laboratory work, and bathing, dressing, and assisting patients in walking and turning. Six tasks that involved more demanding patient care, such as tube feeding and dressing wounds, were ranked as more difficult, and six tasks that involved assembling and using various pieces of complex equipment were rated the most difficult. Research, teaching, supervision, completion of forms, and transporting patients were treated separately as miscellaneous tasks. Although the lists of tasks used in the pilot study were relatively compact, most performers agreed that the listed duties accounted for an overwhelming portion of their workweek. It was therefore concluded that the tasks listed represented a fairly complete and accurate description of the work actually performed.

Significant overlap occurred in tasks performed by LPNs and NAs, even among respondents employed by the same hospital. It was found that 78 percent of the LPNs spent about 25 percent of their time on the six most difficult tasks, while 43 percent of the NAs spent 13 percent of their work time on these same duties. Furthermore, 84 percent of the NAs spent an average of 60 percent of their time performing the easy tasks, while 82 percent of the LPNs spent nearly 50 percent of their time on the very same functions. It is important to realize that the LPN is typically exposed to fifteen or more months of formal training after high school graduation, whereas the NA usually receives only a few weeks of informal, on-the-job training and often lacks a high school diploma.

Despite the rapid increase in the number of laboratory procedures performed per hospital admission, as well as the changes in both technology and skill composition in the hospital laboratory, the time spent on tasks of given difficulty differed little between technicians and technologists in all the laboratory fields studied except cytology (see table 2). In addition, the majority of technicians performed the same tasks as the technologists in their respective fields, despite the technologists' higher level of education.

Of the microbiology, hematology, and biochemistry technologists, 80 percent had at least a bachelor's degree. Only cytotechnologists and blood bank technologists had smaller percentages (67 and 36, respectively). In contrast, most technicians had only twelve to fifteen months of training beyond their high school diplomas. Considering the large overlap in tasks performed, the propriety of current education requirements for effective manpower utilization is questionable.

Approximately 75 percent of physical therapists and physical therapy aides performed the six relatively easy functions, which consumed about 25 and 50 percent of their time, respectively. About 75 percent of the therapists and 50 percent of the aides performed the more difficult tasks, using about 33 percent and 20 percent of their respective work effort. Bachelor's degrees were held by 90 percent of the therapists, whereas 60 percent of the aides had only a high school education and 20 percent had never gone beyond elementary school. Considering a possible increase of over 150 percent in the demand for physical therapists by 1980, some reorganization of responsibilities seems indicated.[7]

If one groups all health employees not holding an undergraduate college degree, there appears to be much similarity in the education of personnel in different occupations performing diverse tasks (see table 3). The high school diploma is usually thought to be a prerequisite for most health occupations, and indeed a large percentage of employees in these occupations were high school graduates. Still, a significant number who lacked this credential had successfully entered the health work force. Thus, a sizable minority of the employees in a number of health occupations could be considered overqualified if the standard of a high school diploma is used. The evidence seems to indicate that there is a real need to develop realistic educational requirements.

Relatively few of the health personnel indicated that their formal education had been a significant influence in preparing them for their current medical functions (see table 4). Occupational or

Table 2. Percent of Workers in Selected Allied Health Occupations Performing Tasks of Specified Difficulty and Percent of Their Time Spent at Those Tasks, in 20 Boston Hospitals, 1968

Occupation	Number of workers interviewed	Easy tasks Percent of workers	Easy tasks Percent of time	Difficult tasks Percent of workers	Difficult tasks Percent of time
Microbiology technologist	8	81.3	31.6	54.0	12.3
Microbiology technician	19	86.0	40.3	65.0	13.1
Hematology technologist	10	97.0	60.0	54.0	22.4
Hematology technician	23	87.0	67.0	35.0	17.4
Cytotechnologist	3	27.7	5.2	55.5	94.8
Cytotechnician	7	47.6	36.2	45.2	63.9
Histotechnologist	5	83.3	69.2	53.3	15.0
Histotechnician	12	88.8	79.3	65.2	11.7
Biochemistry technologist	11	80.3	43.5	72.7	26.7
Biochemistry technician	22	90.1	52.8	71.2	27.2
Blood bank technologist	11	81.8	37.9	80.3	33.0
Blood bank technician	12	84.7	37.1	66.7	46.3

Source: Horowitz and Goldstein, *Hiring Standards for Paramedical Manpower,* pp. 22-26.

Table 3. Percent of Allied Health Workers in 20 Boston Hospitals Completing Specified Years of Schooling and Earning Specified Degrees, by Occupation, 1968

Occupation	Completed 4 years high school	High school diploma[1]	Years of college completed				Associate degree	Bachelor's degree
			2 or less	3	4	5 or more		
Laboratory technician:								
Microbiology	50.0	94.4	33.3	16.7	—	—	5.6	—
Hematology	52.4	100.0	47.6	—	—	—	—	—
Cytology	28.6	71.4	57.1	14.3	—	—	14.3	—
Histology	58.5	83.5	33.3	—	—	8.5	8.5	8.5
Biochemistry	64.0	95.5	31.5	4.5	—	—	4.5	—
Blood bank	58.5	83.5	25.0	8.5	8.5	—	8.5	8.5
Radiation therapist	91.5	100.0	8.5	—	—	—	—	—
X-ray technician	87.9	100.0	12.1	—	—	—	—	—
X-ray developing machine operator[2]	55.5	55.5	—	—	11.1	—	—	11.1
EKG technician	25.0	68.8	43.8	6.3	25.0	—	6.3	25.00
EEG technician[2]	50.0	90.0	30.0	10.0	—	—	—	—
Inhalation therapist[2]	35.3	82.4	35.3	—	5.9	5.9	—	5.9
Licensed practical nurse[2]	85.0	94.0	9.0	—	—	—	—	—
Nurse's aide[2]	57.0	67.0	11.0	—	—	—	—	—

Source: Horowitz and Goldstein, *Hiring Standards for Paramedical Manpower*, tables 9, 51-56, and 86-90.

[1]Includes persons obtaining diploma by attending night school and by passing an equivalency examination, as well as those obtaining it by completing a 4-year daytime high school curriculum.

[2]The following percentages indicate 8 years or less of schooling — 11.1 percent of x-ray developing machine operators, 2.0 percent of licensed practical nurses, and 2.0 percent of nurse's aides. The following percentages indicate 1 to 3 years of high school — 22.2 percent of x-ray developing machine operators, 10.0 percent of EEG technicians, 17.6 percent of inhalation therapists, 4.0 percent of licensed practical nurses, and 30.0 percent of nurse's aides; 5.0 percent of inhalation therapists reported a master's degree.

Table 4. Percent Distribution of Selected Allied Health Workers, Estimates of the Contribution of Different Sources of Learning to Preparation for Current Jobs, in 20 Boston Hospitals, 1968

Occupation	High school	College	Source of Learning Occupational training	On-the-job training	Work experience	Other
Laboratory technician[1]	8.2	10.5	30.0	34.0	16.1	1.1
Microbiology	10.0	19.5	23.3	32.2	16.1	—
Hematology	7.0	10.9	34.5	28.4	15.5	—
Cytology	.8	22.9	27.9	44.5	.8	2.9
Histology	15.4	6.4	22.3	35.5	20.4	—
Biochemistry	6.7	6.1	41.4	29.4	14.1	4.0
Blood Bank	5.4	4.6	17.0	50.8	21.3	—
Nonlaboratory occupations[1]	9.3	4.0	28.0	29.0	30.2	—
Radiation therapist	16.3	8.4	28.4	32.6	14.3	—
X-ray technician	5.5	11.0	30.3	29.7	23.5	—
X-ray developing machine operator	11.3	6.3	1.5	46.5	34.4	—
EKG technician	4.0	8.0	13.7	58.7	15.6	—
EEG technician	13.5	3.0	33.5	35.0	15.0	—
Inhalation therapist	10.0	2.4	27.6	35.6	24.4	—
Licensed practical nurse	11.6	1.3	59.2	29.8	17.7	—
Nurse's aide	7.9	.5	—	31.2	60.4	—
Total, laboratory and nonlaboratory occupations[1]	8.0	6.0	28.3	30.3	26.0	.3

Source: Horowitz and Goldstein, *Hiring Standards for Paramedical Manpower*, tables 12, 63-68, and 96-100.

[1] Weighted average computed from published data for specific occupations.

Note: Detail may not add to 100 percent because of rounding.

professional training was viewed as more important than high school and college combined, and on-the-job training was considered the most important and relevant preparation. On-the-job training and work experience accounted for at least 50 percent of their relevant learning experiences.

In some cases the value placed on formal education by health employees contrasted sharply with the typical training requirements of the institution they worked for. For example, one of the hospitals trained EEG and EKG technicians; the training program required a high school diploma, and candidates with two years of college and a science background were preferred. Impressive as this goal was, it appeared to be unnecessarily high. Less than 50 percent of the EEG technicians and approximately 75 percent of the EKG technicians had gone beyond high school, but only 3 and 8 percent, respectively, indicated that college was helpful preparation for their health positions.

The United States Naval Hospital in Boston, in contrast to the civilian hospitals included in this study, had fewer educational requirements and shorter training requirements. A comparison of the length of training required in the Naval Hospital and the civilian hospitals showed the following: x-ray technicians—twelve months compared with twenty-four months; EEG technicians— four months compared with seven to twelve months; and laboratory assistants—twenty-eight weeks compared with twelve to sixteen months. Despite the fact that navy-trained corpsmen did not meet the formal civilian standards for various specialties, roughly 85 percent of the navy personnel were moonlighting in civilian hospitals in Boston. Furthermore, on the average they were moonlighting for more hours per week than they worked in their regular navy jobs. The obvious demand for navy personnel raises some questions concerning the customary civilian standards of education and training, especially the *amount* of training realistically needed to perform effectively in health care occupations.

The standards that do exist may be the result of either employers' policies or of licensing, certification, and accreditation requirements. The original purpose of licensing was to protect the consumer from fraud and to offer some assurance that health personnel possessed an acceptable degree of competence in their fields. In turn, the licensing process gave the health provider government certification, indicating to the public at large that certain standards had been met. It also gave the provider a greater degree of geographic mobility. Licensing directly limited entrance into the occupation and indirectly had a positive impact on the earning capacity of workers in the profession.

Individual occupational and professional groups have generally taken the initiative in instituting licensing in the health care industry. It would be naive to conclude that professional associations pressuring for licensure are unaware of or unconcerned with the implications of their activities on the supply of personnel. In general, licensing increases the cost of entry to the occupation; produces favorable income effects for the licensees; results in higher age of entry into the field; requires longer periods of schooling than are strictly necessary for acquiring the skills relevant to the job[8]; and protects members of an occupational group from competion by outsiders.

Certification is an alternative to licensure. Members of various health occupations who meet certain standards can be certified. It is important to note that although performers who do not meet the standard are not certified, they can and do perform the same services as those who receive certification. Since the certification process is somewhat less restrictive, it is referred to as permissive licensing.

Although there has been a marked increase in licensing in the health profession, it has had limited impact on actual health practices and consequently on the labor market itself. Enforcement of licensing and certification requirements in a hospital setting is very difficult. When a medical service in a hospital has to be performed, someone—presumably qualified regardless of credentials or occupation—is assigned to perform the job. Overlap in the performance of medical tasks is extensive among health personnel, and the decisions of physicians and supervisors as to who is to perform what medical function are often arbitrary. Various nursing functions are performed by entry-level nurse's aides as well as by licensed practical nurses and by registered nurses. Institutional practices such as these make it difficult for a licensed profession to assume exclusive responsibility for certain functions.

To complicate the matter further, it is not all clear which group performs in the most acceptable fashion—certified personnel, licensed personnel, or entry-level personnel who have had on-the-job training.

An article in the *New England Journal of Medicine* by Ballenger and Estes outlines the alleged disadvantages of the licensure process:

[Licensure] provides no real guarantee of the quality or professional acceptance of the group licensed . . . . It is questionable whether substantial quality control can be exerted by an administrative board having at best only intermittent contacts with the practioners whom it licenses.[9]

If the activities of designated professions are precisely delineated, as required by licensure, a restructuring of medical functions cannot be accomplished without a time-consuming, costly effort to change the licensing laws. If the medical functions remain loosely defined, nonuniform interpretations by certifying boards and legal vagueness are the result. Finally, as new functions emerge through technological and organizational changes, licensed professions—jealously guarding their boundaries—can frustrate reasonable and beneficial changes. This inhibits innovation at a time when innovative changes are needed to contain costs.

Ballenger, a lawyer, and Estes, a physician, are addressing themselves to the licensure of allied health personnel, but their comments can also be applied to their own professions. In particular, the licensing laws governing physicians are obviously the model at which all other allied health personnel look with envy. Once a physician is given a license to practice medicine, it is for life, since the instances of medical licenses being revoked for any reason, justifiable or not, are extremely rare.

Findings and Recommendations

The findings of the *Hiring Standards* study, in conjunction with earnings data, seem to imply that shortages in the allied health professions during 1967-68 existed because of relatively low earnings, a general lack of advancement potential, and job descriptions and hiring standards that tended to encourage educational over-kill rather than preparation relevant to the job. The study's recommendations were aimed at making the education requirements and career structure more realistic:

1. Hospitals should reexamine their whole allied health occupational structure to determine the real job requirements of each occupation.

2. Hospitals should establish hiring standards that are relevant to the tasks performed; educational requirements that are not needed for satisfactory performance should be eliminated.

3. Hospitals should expand their on-the-job training programs for more allied health occupations, and employees should be trained in tasks needed on the job.

4. The educational establishment, including universities, colleges, public school systems, and teaching hospitals, should offer training programs for allied health occupations. Entrance requirements should focus on the skills demanded by the job in order to give as many educationally deprived persons as possible an opportunity to enter the programs.

5. The federal government should reorient its training program under the Manpower Development and Training Act to meet the specific job requirements established by hospitals for these occupations. More such courses should be offered, with a concerted drive to attract disadvantaged workers and school dropouts.

6. Local governments should examine the whole practice of licensing in the allied health occupations, a practice that has tended to exclude school dropouts and the disadvantaged by requiring arbitrary and unnecessary qualification.

7. Wherever possible, hospitals should develop a job promotion ladder, with the necessary training furnished on the job; such a ladder should eliminate dead-end jobs and create advancement opportunities, thereby enabling hospitals to attract better personnel, reduce attrition, and improve the impact of programs for the disadvantaged.

8. Hospitals should coordinate their hiring standards at *some* minimum level that would both provide the quality of service needed and utilize a greater proportion of disadvantaged persons.[10]

In general, these 1968 recommendations are still applicable ten years later.

3

Restructuring Health Occupations

Our 1968 study *Hiring Standards for Paramedical Manpower* apparently confirmed some general knowledge of personnel practices in the health care industry. What was not known was whether individual hospitals would be willing to make the changes necessary for a rationalization of their occupational structures. We were again sponsored by the Employment and Training Administration of the Department of Labor in a research project entitled *Restructuring Paramedical Occupations: A Case Study.*[1] The project ran from June 1969 to November 1971.

The principal objectives of the research project were as follows:

1. To study and analyze the hiring-in requirements and the duties and functions of allied health personnel in a single hospital

2. To recommend changes to restructure occupations and to improve the utilization of manpower in that hospital

3. To evaluate the successes and failures involved in the implementation of the recommendations

4. To measure changes in the quantity and quality of medical services resulting from the implementation of the recommendations and to document the relationship between the changes in services and the specific changes made in hiring-in standards, job duties and functions, and job structure

An additional objective of the project was to study and analyze the problems encountered when a hospital introduces some basic changes in its occupational structure. Such an analysis could help determine whether obstacles to implementation are unique to a specific hospital or are basic to all hospitals. All problems encountered in the implementation of changes were to be recorded in detail. It was assumed that a description of the innovative process in one hospital could have a "demonstration" effect on other hospitals struggling with similar problems and that the findings of this one case study could point up legal, institutional, and other barriers to change that were likely to occur in other hospitals.

Because we were interested in developing recommendations that would be applicable to many hospitals across the nation, the initial step was to find a hospital that was as representative as possible of others in the United States. In addition, the hospital's administrators had to be willing to cooperate in this research project. The following criteria were developed for the selection of a hospital:

1. A hospital of modest size with a minimum of two hundred beds

2. A hospital with progressive and forceful administration

3. A hospital administration with a genuine interest in organizational efficiency, equitable employment opportunities, and, most importantly, the delivery of quality service to the public for a reasonable and equitable cost

After a considerable search we found a hospital that met our criteria in The Cambridge Hospital, Cambridge, Massachusetts, which was under the supervision of Dr. James Hartgering, commissioner of Health, Hospitals, and Welfare for the city of Cambridge.

We should not leave the impression that, because the administration of The Cambridge Hospital and several professional organizations, unions, and physicians cooperated in this project, there was or is now complete harmony at that institution. The Cambridge Hospital faces problems similar to those of most hospitals in this country, since it is a city hospital, many of its problems are compounded. Unlike those in many hospitals, The Cambridge Hospital administrators were willing to cooperate in the study and from the start they demonstrated an interest in implementing recommended changes.

The changes that were made at The Cambridge Hospital during this period must be attributed principally to the cooperation of the commissioner of Health, to changes in the composition of the medical staff of the hospital, and to the positive attitude of nursing and administrative personnel. Without their willingness to experiment with change, the study's recommendations, good or bad, would never have received a test. The presence of the study group at the hospital and its interviews and conversations with numerous staff persons undoubtedly provided some motivation for implementing changes.

Methodology Used in the Project

1. In-depth interviews were held with supervisors of the thirteen health occupation categories included in the study in order to elicit a complete and exact list of assigned tasks and responsibilities of the employees under their jurisdiction. (The terms *function* and *task* are used interchangeably throughout this study.) Table 5 indicates, for each occupation, the number interviewed, the total number of persons employed, and the percentage interviewed.

2. In-depth interviews (ranging in time from one and a half to two and a half hours) were held with several health employees in each of the occupational categories to elicit a complete and exact list of performed duties, tasks, and responsibilities.

3. These two independent job descriptions were then compared. If one included a task or an element of a task not described by the other, it was checked (for example, "The hematology technician under your jurisdiction states that he operates an autoclave; you, his supervisor, did not list this task in our interview. Does he or does he not use the autoclave?")

4. After analyzing and cross-checking the results for each occupational category, the tasks were then compared with the lists of functions compiled in the pilot study, *Hiring Standards for Paramedical Manpower*. The listed functions in that study were the result of detailed interviews with approximately four hundred and fifty performers and one hundred and fifty supervisors, specialists, administrators, and pathologists.

5. To be certain that each interviewer and each performer would interpret tasks in the same way, each task was defined in terms of the elements of every function. This proved to be an enormous project. With the aid of private consultants and senior nursing and administrative personnel at The Cambridge Hospital, every task was defined in detail. The interviewer then had an accurate description of each task.

6. All the functions for each of the occupations studied were ranked in order of difficulty, using criteria such as the level of practical experience and educational exposure necessary to perform the task. The ranking was completed by the researchers with the assistance of supervisory personnel (both nursing and medical) at

Table 5. Number and Percentage of Personnel Interviewed by Occupation

Occupation	Number interviewed	Total number employed	Percentage interviewed
Registered nurse	45	51	88.2
Licensed practical nurse	10	17	58.8
Nurse's aide	28	31	90.3
Orderly	8	8	100.0
Ward secretary	6	9	66.7
Surgical technician	7	8	87.5
Psychiatric attendant	7	7	100.0
X-ray technician	12	12	100.0
EKG technician	1	1	100.0
Inhalation therapy technician	4	4	100.0
Neighborhood health worker	1	1	100.0
Laboratory technician:			
1. Hematology technician	2	2	100.0
2. Blood bank technician	2	3	66.7
3. Bacteriology technician	2	2	100.0
4. Cytology technician	1	1	100.0
5. Histology technician	2	2	100.0
6. Urinalysis and parasitology technician	1	1	100.0
7. Chemistry	2	2	100.0
Administrative and supervisory personnel	38	42	90.5
Total	179	204	87.7

Source: CMMS Survey

The Cambridge Hospital and at several other medical centers. A sample of the performers was also asked to aid in this ranking.

7. The interview formats were then prepared, and all responses were obtained and recorded by the interviewer. No respondent was asked to fill out a questionnaire. Instead, each was shown the list of functions and asked if they represented 95 percent of the tasks he or she performed over an average workweek. Significant additions to the interview format were made in only two areas—the psychiatry department and the ward secretaries.

8. Because of the possibility that some performers might tend to exaggerate their own authority and responsibility, observations of approximately 50 percent of the sample were made. These observations were made by a graduate registered nurse and a research assistant. At times, one performer was observed for a period of four to five hours. However, in most cases, two or three performers in one ward or unit were observed by both the registered nurse and a research assistant for a period of four or five hours. Approximately three hundred hours of observations were conducted during a two-month period. The graduate registered nurse was an outside consultant to the project, not an employee or former employee of the hospital.

9. Because it was difficult for each performer to estimate the amount of time he or she spent in the average week on each of the more than sixty functions, a code was developed (indicated below) to make the selection somewhat easier and more accurate.

Time spent/week (40 hours)	Percent
Under 30 minutes	Less than 1
30 minutes-2 hours	1-5
2 hours-4 hours	6-10
4 hours-6 hours	11-15
6 hours-10 hours	16-25
Over 10 hours	Greater than 25

In estimating time spent on each function, performers were asked to make their estimates in hours or percentages, whichever they found easier. Any performer who estimated "over ten hours" or "greater than 25 percent" was asked to be more specific (for example, "Would you estimate twenty hours out of forty hours or 50 percent of your time?"). A specific number of hours over ten or a specific percentage of time over 25 percent was finally obtained from each performer.

10. Table 6 averages all performers' time, whether they performed the function or not, and therefore should add up to 100 percent. We assumed that there was not disproportionate individual bias and adjusted proportionately the amount of time spent on each group of functions so that the total added up to 100 percent. Group 6 was not adjusted since lunch and breaks are specifically allocated periods of time.

The functions were separated into six groups, ranked from easiest to most difficult:

Group	Functions
1	1-18
2	19-30
3	31-47
4	48-63
5	64-69
6	Lunch and breaks

It was impossible to differentiate the degree of difficulty of functions within a group, but we could differentiate between groups. No comparison was made using groups 5 and 6 since group 5 comprised several different departments (pediatrics and labor and delivery) and group 6 represented lunch and breaks.

Analysis of Data

Almost all persons interviewed in the four occupations (RNs, LPNs, NAs, and orderlies) performed the easiest functions. For example, the task of straightening and cleaning the patient's immediate furniture was performed by 91 percent of the RNs; 100 percent of the LPNs; 96 percent of the NAs; and 100 percent of the orderlies. The RNs and LPNs spent a larger percentage of time than NAs and orderlies on this easy function, RNs and LPNs spending 7.5 and 9.2 percent, respectively, NAs 6 percent and orderlies 4.9 percent.

Going to a more difficult function, demanding more skill and training, we found that the function "discontinuing I.V. service" was performed by all the LPNs, almost all the RNs, and slightly more than half of the NAs and orderlies. For those who performed this difficult function, the following average time was spent on it: 5.1 percent by RNs; 5.1 percent by LPNs; 1.9 percent by NAs; and 2.7 percent by orderlies.

The groupings in table 6 indicate that (for general nursing) on the simplest functions (1-18) RNs spent 24.7 percent of their time; LPNs spent 31.5 percent of their time; NAs spent 40.8 percent of their time; and orderlies spent 40.8 percent of their time. If we go to the more difficult functions (ones that are not supervisory), such as group 3 (31-47), we see that on these functions RNs spent 20.3 percent of their time; LPNs spent 22.5 percent of their time; NAs spent 6.4 percent of their time; and orderlies spent 15.6 percent of their time.

From these statistical data the following conclusions were reached:

1. There was indeed a great deal of overlap in the performance cf various functions regardless of the degree of difficulty and the educational exposure, formal or otherwise, of various categories of paramedical personnel (RNs, LPNs, NAs, and orderlies) at The Cambridge Hospital.

2. Although the more difficult functions tended to be performed more by personnel with higher levels of professional training and knowledge, the lesser-skilled health employee did perform these functions occasionally.

3. The more highly skilled persons in this sample spent large blocks of their time on functions they themselves and most other authorities considered well below their technical capabilities.

4. All four of these health occupations (RNs, LPNs, NAs, and orderlies) performed most of their high-level functions during shifts other than the day shift. This was especially true of the LPNs, NAs, and orderlies. During the shift from 11 P.M. to 7 A.M., RNs, LPNs, NAs, and orderlies were called upon to perform functions that only physicians or RNs would normally perform during the day.

The above analysis of nursing occupations covers more than 60 percent of the occupations of interest to The Cambridge Hospital study. A similar analysis was made for the other occupations and can be found in the original complete report of the study, *Restructuring Paramedical Occupations.*

Table 6. Average Percent of Time Spent on Six Groups of Functions by Registered Nurses, Licensed Practical Nurses, Nurse's Aides, and Orderlies[1]

I. General nursing[2]

Groups of functions	Functions	RN	LPN	Nurse's aid	Orderly
(Ranked from easiest to most difficult)					
1	(1-18)	24.7	31.5	40.8	40.8
2	(19-30)	26.3	28.2	38.2	26.1
3	(31-47)	20.3	22.5	6.4	15.6
4	(48-63)	16.6	8.8	3.0	3.1
5	(64-69)	3.1	0.1	2.7	5.2
6	Lunch & break	8.8	8.8	8.8	8.8

II. Surgical unit

Groups of functions	Functions	RN	LPN	Nurse's aide	Orderly
(Ranked from easiest to most difficult)					
1	(1-18)	26.1	28.0	39.4	36.7
2	(19-30)	31.3	33.7	41.9	29.1
3	(31-47)	22.8	17.2	7.9	16.5
4	(48-63)	14.7	12.0	1.6	1.5
5	(64-69)	0.8	0.3	0.3	7.5
6	Lunch & break	8.8	8.8	8.8	8.8

III. *Medical unit*

Groups of functions	*Functions*	RN	LPN	Nurse's aide	Orderly
(Ranked from easiest to most difficult)					
1	(1-18)	23.4	27.4	36.3	39.0
2	(19-30)	27.4	28.9	47.2	27.7
3	(31-47)	20.6	28.6	4.5	15.2
4	(48-63)	18.8	6.2	0.5	3.8
5	(64-69)	0.8	—	2.7	5.6
6	Lunch & break	8.8	8.8	8.8	8.8

IV. *Pediatrics unit*

Groups of functions	*Functions*	RN	LPN	Nurse's aide	Orderly
(Ranked from easiest to most difficult)					
1	(1-18)	32.8	42.9	51.7	—
2	(19-30)	23.7	21.5	24.2	—
3	(31-47)	17.6	12.7	7.4	—
4	(48-63)	12.6	12.0	4.8	—
5	(64-69)	4.9	2.0	3.1	—
6	Lunch & break	8.8	8.8	8.8	—

See footnotes at end of table.

Table 6 (cont.)

V. Labor and delivery unit	RN	LPN	Nurse's aide	Orderly
Groups of functions — Functions				
(Ranked from easiest to most difficult)				
1 (1–18)	19.4	—	35.4	—
2 (19–30)	15.4	—	25.9	—
3 (31–47)	17.3	—	7.5	—
4 (48–63)	19.6	—	6.7	—
5 (64–69)	19.5	—	15.7	—
6 Lunch & break	8.8	—	8.8	—

VI. Emergency unit	RN	LPN	Nurse's aide	Orderly
Groups of functions — Functions				
(Ranked from easiest to most difficult)				
1 (1–18)	—	39.1	—	43.2
2 (19–30)	—	23.6	—	21.4
3 (31–47)	—	20.2	—	20.5
4 (48–63)	—	7.8	—	5.9
5 (64–69)	—	0.4	—	—
6 Lunch & break	—	8.8	—	8.8

VII. *Outpatient department*

Groups of functions	Functions	RN	LPN	Nurse's aide	Orderly
(Ranked from easiest to most difficult)					
1	(1-18)	26.5	—	49.5	—
2	(19-30)	24.3	—	30.5	—
3	(31-47)	21.3	—	10.2	—
4	(48-63)	17.0	—	0.9	—
5	(64-69)	2.0	—	—	—
6	Lunch & break	8.8	—	8.8	—

Source: CMMS Survey

[1]This table is the average of all performers' time whether they perform the function or not; therefore, it should add up to 100 percent except for roundings. These figures were adjusted proportionately to add up to 100 percent because we felt that there was no reason to believe that disproportionate bias occurred in estimation of time for each group as a whole. Group 6 was not adjusted because this is a specifically allocated period of time.

[2]This section is a summary of all specific units, i.e., surgical, medical, pediatrics, labor and delivery, emergency, and outpatient departments. The RN column also includes ICU, recovery room, and "floats."

Recommendations to The Cambridge Hospital

The objectives of the health resources of any city should include the following:

1. To minimize the discomfort and costs of hospitalization, preventive medicine information should be disseminated through the city's public health service and the city's medical facilities.

2. Once a patient is admitted to the hospital, the principal aim should be to make this stay as comfortable, brief, inexpensive, and successful as medical technology and human patience can achieve.

The city of Cambridge had recently replaced the main hospital complex with a $12 million facility, and the city's objectives did include those listed above. However, there were no indications that any attention was given to the possibility of eliminating dead-end, low-paying jobs or of creating occupational ladders for health personnel.

Our project was concerned with the problem of operating a hospital efficiently and humanely by utilizing its manpower in the most effective manner possible. Based on an analysis of the information collected, a number of recommendations were made to The Cambridge Hospital in January 1971.

Recommendation 1

The hospital had no personnel director, and personnel structure was extremely informal and haphazard. When a supervisor, physician, director of nursing, or the hospital director had a request or saw a need for a new position or a replacement, each acted as a personnel administrator. Four or five separate files existed in the hospital for each employee. No formal and systematic review of employee performance existed. The precious and costly time of many hospital employees was spent in repetitious and, quite often, unproductive personnel work. When employees had problems or questions, they quite often went for advice to the persons they knew best and frequently the answers were wrong or misleading.

Our recommendation was to establish a permanent personnel office, at the hospital, headed by a personnel director. No additional funds were required to set up this office and position, since there were at least three unrelated positions in the hospital that had personnel responsibilities. The personnel director would maintain the only complete set of records for each employee in the hospital. The director would have a voice in, if not control over, the following:

1. Setting hiring standards in conjunction with supervisors of the appropriate departments

2. Overseeing conduct of personnel

3. Orienting new personnel

4. Coordinating in-service and on-the-job training (OJT) programs

5 Securing performance reports at least once each year on each employee

6. Making the initial contact with all prospective employees (final approval of any employee would be made by the supervisor or physician for whom she or he would work)

7. Keeping all employees of the hospital informed of their rights, privileges, and obligations

Recommendation 2

Lines of authority were not well known nor were they publicized in the hospital. It was recommended that a formal organization chart for The Cambridge Hospital be developed.

Recommendation 3

The study data indicated that various categories of health personnel at The Cambridge Hospital were underutilized and numerous functions were misallocated. The most frequently mentioned reasons for these conditions were tradition and the unwillingness of supervisory personnel to allocate more sensitive and responsible functions to persons considered untrained or insufficiently trained.

In some instances the concern on the part of supervisory personnel appeared to be justified. On the other hand, in many instances responsible and sensitive functions were being performed by nurse's aides, orderlies, inhalation therapy technicians, surgical technicians, psychiatric attendants, and corpsmen-types at the hospital. The question was how we could eliminate the apprehension of supervisory personnel while granting to all categories of health personnel responsibility commensurate with their present or post-training capabilities. The belief was that the best solution would be threefold: (1) the establishment of three new health occupations at The Cambridge Hospital, (2) the restructuring of four existing occupations at the hospital, and (3) the establishment of formal training programs for the three new occupations and four existing occupations.

The new health occupations recommended were *nursing assistant, medical assistant* (medics), and *physician's assistant.* Persons employed in these occupations could be male or female.

The nursing assistant would be trained to perform some of the moderately sophisticated functions previously performed by LPNs and RNs and some of the more sophisticated functions performed by NAs. The minimum entrance requirement for the nursing assistant training program was to be the equivalent of a five-week training program as a nurse's aide.

The medical assistants, including corpsmen-types, would be divorced from the nursing department and placed in the department of medicine. The medical assistants (and physician's assistants) would be under the direct control of the medical staff who would be responsible for their training and supervision. After their formal training, medical assistants would be in a position to aid substantially the medical staff in functions previously performed by physicians. The minimum entrance requirements for the medical assistants would be the completion of a nursing assistant program.

The physician's assistant would be one level above the medical assistant. After being exposed to a two-year training program, the physician's assistant would be in a position to assist substantially the physician in some of the more sophisticated functions traditionally performed by physicians alone. Specific training programs for physician's assistant had recently been instituted in several states with promising results. The suggestion was made that the "Medex" training program at the University of Washington or the "Physician's Associate Program" at Duke University be used as a basis for training the physician's assistant.

In order to provide a better quality of medical care within the hospital and to establish these three new occupational categories, recommendations were made to *restructure* the positions of nurse's aide, ward secretary, licensed practical nurse, and registered nurse. The specific changes in functions for each of these occupations were detailed in the complete study. In summary, the recommendation was to downgrade the nurse's aides and upgrade the ward secretaries, licensed practical nurses, and registered nurses.

The seven training programs recommended were the following:

1. *Nursing aides:* a five-week training program for entry-level personnel, consisting of one hour of lecture and six hours of supervised work per day. It makes little sense in terms of delivery of quality medical care to allow entry-level personnel to wander about the hospital with no exposure to basic policies and medical procedures within their occupation. Entry requirements for this position should allow for inclusion of those with no previous medical training and no high school diploma.

2. *Nursing assistants:* a twelve-week training program for persons completing the nurse's aide program or its equivalent consisting of one hour of lecture and six hours of supervised work per day.

3. *Medical assistants:* a twelve-week training program for persons completing the nursing assistant program or its equivalent, consisting of one hour of lecture and six hours of supervised work per day.

4. *Physician's assistants:* a two-year training program for persons completing the medical assistant program or its equivalent.

5. *Ward secretaries:* an eight-week training program for entry-level personnel with basic reading and writing skills. The program should consist of one hour of lecture and six hours of supervised work per day. In the past, orientation for ward secretaries had

been minimal. A large majority of this group felt a definite need for training in their present function. RNs, LPNs, and NAs were spending considerable time on non-nursing functions that should have been assigned to ward secretaries. Head nurses and supervisors indicated a reluctance to allow ward secretaries more non-nursing, administrative responsibilities. Very often, the lack of experience and training of ward secretaries was given as the reason for this reluctance. An eight-week training program for ward secretaries seemed appropriate.

6. *Licensed practical nurses:* an ongoing, in-service education program, consisting of one class hour per week.

7. *Registered Nurses:* an ongoing, in-service education program, consisting of one class hour per week.

In light of the new techniques and tools being developed, RNs and LPNs who had no ongoing, in-service education soon found their previous training inadequate. It was recommended that the seven training programs be started, in selected wards or units, simultaneously and as soon as possible. The training program was to be designed to extend knowledge and to give assurance to those already performing high-level functions in their respective fields. In this way, each performer would be accepted in his or her department with a degree of confidence that did not exist among superiors and supervisors at the time this recommendation was made.

A small committee of qualified persons was to shoulder the responsibility of sifting through all candidates to determine their qualifications and acceptability. The study group saw no need to place any formal educational requirements on a prospective applicant. Each applicant was to be judged on his or her own merits and capabilities.

Recommendation 4

An immediate efforts was to be made to decrease the time RNs spent on group 1 functions (functions 1-18, table 6). RNs had reported that they performed all the functions in group 1 and spent 24.7 percent of their time on them. Observations made during the study period substantiated this. These functions could be readily assigned to either nurse's aides or nursing assistants. No additional training of other health personnel at the hospital was required to effect this reassignment.

Recommendation 5

To motivate personnel to undertake and complete training programs, some monetary incentive had to be offered, in addition to a certificate and a title. It was recommended that a salary differential be established for those who completed training and were advanced to a higher position.

Recommendation 6

It was recommended that training programs be well publicized throughout the hospital and qualified health personnel be encouraged to enroll. Absolutely no pressure was to be used to enroll candidates.

Recommendation 7

The interview format used in this study was to be used as a basis for a detailed job description of each of the thirteen occupations. (One may note that the same list of functions was constructed for RNs, LPNs, NAs, and orderlies. This was done to determine the overlap of functions. The degree of responsibility was to be stated explicitly in the job descriptions.)

Recommendation 8

It was recommended that the job category of orderly be eliminated. The functions normally performed by the orderly could be done easily by nurse's aides or nursing assistants.

Recommendation 9

It was recommended that periodic updating on radiological techniques be a permanent practice at the hospital. A minimum of one hour per month was to be set aside in which the radiologist could present new techniques to the technicians.

Recommendation 10

The sole EKG technician at the hospital was employed for thirty-seven hours per week, and there was an obvious need for increased coverage in this area. In-service education programs for RNs and LPNs should include EKG training. It was recommended that the training programs for the nursing assistant, medical assistant, and physician's assistant include this type of training.

Recommendation 11

There was only one neighborhood health worker (NHW) under the jurisdiction of The Cambridge Hospital, and her work did appear to aid RNs and public health nurses at the center. It was recommended that additional NHWs be used at the two new centers, provided that meaningful functions could be prescribed.

Recommendation 12

It was recommended that the unstructured OJT program in inhalation therapy be improved. Experience with navy corpsmen at the United States Naval Medical Center indicated that a three-year, full-time program for the inhalation therapy technician was unnecessary. Trainees in inhalation therapy were to be encouraged to enroll in a more formal program, similar to one offered by the United States Navy.

Recommendation 13

A private laboratory originally performed routine chemistry, hematology, and esoteric tests for The Cambridge Hospital. During the study period The Cambridge Hospital laboratory, under the direction of its new pathologist, began to perform all hematology work in addition to some of the chemistry tests. This turnabout occurred because the hospital was in a position to do the work in the same time as, or less, and for the same price as, or less, than the private laboratory: the floor space allocated to the hospital laboratory had recently been doubled, and the new pathologist had purchased or leased all the automated equipment he thought necessary.

The pathologists who were consultants for the study indicated that a 200-bed hospital, like The Cambridge Hospital, was not large enough to maximize the use of an efficiently run laboratory. However, there were several hospitals in the immediate area of The Cambridge Hospital that maintained laboratories without the services of a full-time pathologist.

The recommendation was made that The Cambridge Hospital laboratory actively seek the laboratory work of Holy Ghost Hospital (one block away) with 290 beds, recently renamed Youville Hospital) and Sancta Maria Hospital (one mile away with 124 beds), neither of which had a full-time pathologist or adequate laboratory facilities. If The Cambridge Hospital laboratory did obtain the additional laboratory work, it would then be feasible to restructure the laboratory occupations.

Status of the Recommendations

The hierarchy in general nursing at The Cambridge Hospital and at most other hospitals in the United States, whether they be governmental, private, nonprofit, or proprietary, appears to be:

Group A	1. Nurse's aide
	2. Orderly
Group B	3. **Licensed practical nurse**
	4. Registered nurse; graduate registered nurse
Group C	5. Head nurse
	6. Nurse supervisor
	7. Director of nursing
Group D	8. Interns
	9. Residents
	10. Chiefs of medicine

With few exceptions, there is no vertical mobility between groups. Should a nurse's aide or an orderly wish to become an LPN, his or her previous training and experience cannot be credited towards the requirements of the higher occupation. Should an LPN wish to become a registered nurse or attain any of the occupations in group C, her previous training and experience are of no formal value. The LPN must start from the beginning at the traditional school of nursing in order to earn her degree as a registered nurse or graduate registered nurse. Should a person in group C have the ability and desire to become a physician, the person is given no credit for previous on-the-job or formal training experience. (There are several programs in the United States that do give advanced credit to LPNs who wish to become RNs. One such program has recently been started at Northeastern University; however, it is very limited—fifteen students. In general such programs are full time and require the participants to give up their jobs.)

Our findings in this study led to the conclusion that this lack of vertical mobility resulted in inefficient use of medical manpower. Specific recommendations to The Cambridge Hospital were aimed at facilitating vertical mobility:

1. An increased use of lower-level personnel, such as nurse's aides and nursing assistants, to complement and, to a certain extent, supplant the use of RNs and LPNs on lower-level functions

2. A restructuring of the jobs of RNs and LPNs, so they would not be asked to perform the lower-level functions

3. In-service training that would allow nurse's aides to advance to the position of nursing assistant

4. In-service training that would allow a nursing assistant to rise to the position of medical assistant

5. In-service training that would allow a medical assistant to rise to the position of physician's assistant

In effect, the recommendations included a new occupational ladder (parallel to the traditional occupational hierarchy of the hospital) aimed at more efficient utilization of the talents of various categories of health personnel. This occupational ladder would allow for the transfer of training and experience by establishing the following occupational hierarchy:

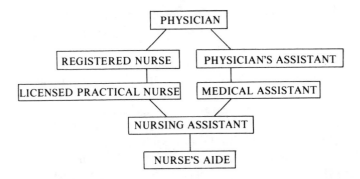

A person with desire and ability could follow the left-hand track by leaving his or her position and starting formal training all over again in order to reach successive steps. Alternatively, one could follow the right-hand track and continue at his or her job while receiving in-service training; this would mean no loss of income and no duplication of formal training.

As of August 1971, the status of the study group's thirteen formal recommendations was as follows:

1. A hospital personnel director was to be requested from the city of Cambridge by the hospital, and a personnel department was to be established.

2. The hospital administration had accepted an organizational chart to be used in structuring future staffing policy.

3. An in-service training program was scheduled to begin in September 1971 to upgrade nurse's aides to the new occupation of nursing assistant. The position of physician's assistant had been established in the medical department of the hospital and three former corpsmen were receiving in-service training for this new occupation. The Cambridge Hospital had given letters of intent to employ the physician's assistants who successfully completed the eighteen-month training program at Northeastern University. In-service education programs had been instituted, as recommended, for RNs and LPNs.

4. RNs were performing fewer group 1 functions ("easy" functions), and a significant number of nurse's aides had been hired to perform these tasks.

5. Approval had been given to provide increases in salary for all those paramedical personnel who successfully complete any in-service, upgrading program.

6. The AFSCME union, representing the nurse's aides and orderlies, had strongly endorsed the proposal for training and upgrading health employees.

7. The hospital administration had agreed to combine this study's detailed interview formats with the less detailed job descriptions arrived at by the hospital's job description committee.

8. Orderlies at the hospital were being phased out.

9. The radiological technicians were attending weekly conferences of surgeons to receive explanations of new procedures and techniques.

10. A number of various health employees (RNs, LPNs) had been exposed to training in the use of EKG equipment.

11. An additional neighborhood health worker had been employed and several others were to be employed in the fall of 1972.

12. The inhalation therapy technicians were exposed to occasional lectures on techniques by the department head. However, no formal, in-service training program had been instituted.

13. The hospital's laboratory had actively sought the laboratory work of neighborhood institutions, and this effort had been successful.

Between September 1969 and June 1971 the following job requirements were changed:

1. The requirement of a high school education for nurse's aides was dropped.

2. Specialized practical experience for a hematology laboratory specialist was reduced from two years to one.

3. Psychiatric attendants no longer needed a high school education.

4. Entry requirements for all paramedical personnel included in this study were reviewed by the newly formed job description committee.

Over the two-year period 1968-1970, hospital costs and utilization at The Cambridge Hospital changed as follows:

1. A 19.7 percent increase in bed complement
2. A 38 percent increase in inpatient days
3. A reduction of the average length of stay from 9.6 to 9.3 days
4. A 34 percent increase in outpatient clinic visits
5. A reduction of the hospital's loss as a percent of expenses from 23 percent to 4.3 percent

The changes in employment of health personnel at the hospital from 1969 to 1971 are shown in table 7. A substantial change occurred in the distribution of RNs, LPNs, nurse's aides, orderlies, and ward secretaries employed in general nursing between 1969 and 1971. Over this period, the number of orderlies decreased from 14.5 to 3 full-time equivalents. The number of RNs increased by only 6.7 percent, while nurse's aides experienced the largest percentage increase — 70.9 percent. During these two years the hospital doubled its number of laboratory personnel. In addition, there was a substantial increase in the number of psychiatric attendants, from 6 in 1969 to 11 in 1971.

Table 8 shows salary scales at The Cambridge Hospital for various health occupations for 1969 and 1971. These figures were used to calculate the general nursing wage bill shown on Table 9.

One can legitimately ask what has been the financial impact of the significant change in the staffing pattern in general nursing, which now uses a greater percentage of personnel with less formal training and few license requirements. If general nursing personnel in 1971 were still distributed according to the 1969 pattern, the wage bill (using the midpoint of the 1971 salary ranges) would have amounted to $27,466.23 (table 9, column J). The 1971 weekly wage bill was calculated using the 1971 (FTE) personnel distribution and the midpoint of the 1971 salary ranges (table 9, column I). This wage bill amounted to $26,805.81. A comparison of these two wage bills (columns I and J, table 9) indicates that, as a result of the structural personnel changes from 1969 to June 1971, the wage bill was 2.5 percent lower.

Table 10 shows the changes in the mortality rate and the infant mortality rate at the hospital for 1965-1971, the years when changes in wage and occupational structures were occurring. We are not drawing the conclusion that the changes in hospital costs and utilization, in wage bills and in mortality rates were the direct results of the recommendations adopted by the hospital. However, all the changes can be considered beneficial, and at a minimum one can conclude that the adoption of our recommendations did not lead to a deterioration of efficiency or of quality of service in the hospital.

Table 7. Number and Percent of Persons and Percentage Change in Various Paramedical Occupations Employed at The Cambridge Hospital — 1969, 1971

	October 1969		June 1971		Percentage change
Occupations	Number	Percent	Number	Percent	
General Nursing:					
RN	67	47.0	71.5	40.	+ 6.7
LPN	20	14.0	33.5	19.	+ 67.5
NA	31	21.7	53	30.	+ 70.9
Orderly	14.5	10.1	3	1.7	–383.3
Ward secretary	10	7.0	14	8.0	+ 40.0
General nursing subtotal	142.5	100.0	175.0	100.0	+ 22.8
Laboratory:					
General lab technician	11	73.3	14.5	49.2	+ 31.8
Lab specialist (senior technician): chemistry bacteriology, cytology, blood bank supervisor	2	13.3	4	13.6	+100.0
Lab specialist: hematology, histology	1	6.7	2	6.8	+100.0
Clinical lab supervisor	1	6.7	2	6.8	+100.0
Medical technologist, MT (ASCP)	0	—	7	23.7	Not relevant
Laboratory subtotal	15	100.0	29.5	100.0	+ 96.6
X-ray technician	12	—	11	—	- 9.1
Head x-ray technician	1	—	1	—	—
EKG technician	1	—	1	—	—
Inhalation therapy technician	4	—	5	—	+ 25.0
Surgical technician	8	—	7	—	- 14.3
Neighborhood health worker	1	—	2	—	+100.0
Psychiatric attendant	6	—	11	—	+ 83.3
Physician's assistant	0	—	3	—	Not relevant
Total Full-time equivalent (FTE)	190.5		245.5		+ 28.9

Source: CMMS Survey

Table 8. Weekly Salary Scales at The Cambridge Hospital — 1969, 1971

Occupation	1969 Weekly salary			1971 Weekly salary		
	Minimum	Maximum	Midpoint	Minimum	Maximum	Midpoint
Head nurse	$152.31	$194.69	$170.50	$181.31	$213.15	$206.23
RN	141.73	184.04	162.89	168.74	218.59	193.67
LPN	122.00	146.00	134.00	144.94	173.45	159.20
Nurse's aide	86.25	92.02	89.14	102.06	113.65	107.87
Orderly	94.52	100.67	97.60	111.84	125.03	118.44
Ward secretary	86.25	92.02	89.14	102.06	109.35	105.71
Surgical technician	100.00	115.00	107.50	118.80	136.62	127.71
Psychiatric attendant	122.00	146.00	134.00	144.94	173.45	159.20
X-ray technician	115.19	126.73	120.96	136.87	150.57	143.72
EKG technician	100.77	110.00	105.39	119.73	130.64	125.19
Inhalation therapist[1]	134.61	146.15	140.38	159.92	173.62	166.77
Inhalation technician[1]	105.77	117.30	111.54	125.65	139.35	132.50
Lab technicians (chiefs) Bacteriology Hematology Chemistry Cytology	132.40	143.94	138.17	157.32	171.03	164.18
Lab technician	115.38	126.92	121.15	137.07	150.57	143.82
Medical technologist[2]				162.00		
Physician's assistant[3]	122.00	146.00	134.00	144.94	173.45	159.20

Source: CMMS Survey

[1]Position was established in 1969.

[2]Position was established in 1970. The salary range for medical technologists has not yet been established. All technologists employed in 1971 were being paid at the rate of $162.00 per week.

[3]One corpsman was employed as a medical technician in the department of nursing during the latter part of 1969. It was not until 1971 that the group of corpsmen was transferred to the department of medicine and given the title of physician's assistant.

Table 9. General Nursing Wage Bill Comparisons 1969 and 1971, at the Cambridge Hospital

	Number of personnel (FTE)		Per cent		Midpoint of weekly Salary		1971 Total employment allocated according to % distribution of 1969 employment	1969 Weekly wage bill (using 1969 employment and 1969 salary)	1971 Weekly wage bill (using 1971 employment and 1969 salary)	Calculated wage bill for 1971, assuming occupation distribution of 1969
	1969	1971	1969	1971	1969	1971				
	A	B	C	D	E	F	G	H (Column AxE)	I (Column BxF)	J (Column FxG)
RN head nurse	6	6	4.2	3.4	$173.50	$206.23	7.4	$ 1,041.00	$ 1,237.38	$ 1,526.10
RN	61	65.5	42.8	37.4	162.89	193.67	74.9	9,936.29	12,685.39	14,505.88
LPN	20	33.5	14.0	19.1	134.00	159.20	24.6	2,680.50	5,333.20	3,916.32
NA	31	53	21.7	30.3	89.14	107.86	38.1	2,763.34	5,716.58	4,109.47
Orderly	14.5	3	10.1	1.7	97.60	118.44	17.8	1,415.20	353.32	2,108.23
Ward secretary	10	14	7.0	8.0	89.14	105.71	12.3	891.40	1,479.94	1,300.23
Total	142.5	175.0	100.0	100.0			175.1	$18,727.73	$26,805.81	$27,466.23

Source: CMMS Survey

Table 10. Mortality Rate and Infant Mortality Rate at The Cambridge Hospital, 1965-1971

Year	Mortality rate: percentage of all patients discharged	Mortality rate: percentage of all newborns discharged
1965	5.4	2.5
1966	5.5	2.1
1967	5.3	0.9
1968	5.2	1.7
1969	5.8	2.2
1970	3.6	1.7
1971 January 1 to May 30	3.5	1.0

Source: CMMS Survey

Conclusions

In summary, the use of The Cambridge Hospital facilities increased, and the quality of medical care probably increased, at a time when there had been a disproportionate increase in the use of health personnel with little formal training. The following general conclusions were drawn from this research experience:

1. Hiring-in standards at The Cambridge Hospital were unnecessarily high. Employees with less than the specified required experience and training were found to be sufficiently competent to perform functions of a different nature, not commonly associated with entry-level occupations.

2. Those health employees with more sophisticated training and experience (that is , RNs, LPNs, ex-corpsmen) were found to be underutilized. A reshuffling of their functions, which eliminated "easy" tasks, led to a more efficient utilization of their training and experience.

3. The restructuring of health occupations can lead to greater hospital efficiency, the elimination of possible shortages of health personnel, and the minimization of dead-end, entry-level jobs.

4. A liberalization of hiring-in requirements and the establishment of vertical mobility (with in-service training) could make possible greater utilization of minority and disadvantaged groups.

5. Realistic career ladders are possible once the traditional hospital hierarchy has been short-circuited. For example, in-

service education and training for nursing assistants, medical assistants, and physician's assistants can provide entry-level personnel with attainable upward mobility.

6. The end result of successful restructuring of health occupations could mean a more efficient health care delivery system, that is, increased quality and quantity.

7. Restructuring the occupations of health personnel should begin with physicians. Unless their functions are clearly delineated and perhaps modified, it is somewhat difficult to define and restructure the remaining functions that can be performed more efficiently by the other health occupations.

8. Operational statistics during the period 1968-1970 indicated a substantial increase in the utilization of the hospital's facilities. At the same time, the day-to-day functioning of the hospital had become more hectic. Because administrative problems frequently arise over the efficient utilization of manpower, administrators must have greater leeway in utilizing hospital manpower.

9. The time available to measure and evaluate the changes in the hospital resulting from the implementation of the recommendations appeared short. Such changes take time, and many of the results, as measured by the delivery of service, could not become apparent until a year or two after the changes had been made.

In our final report to the Employment and Training Administration, we made the following general recommendations:

1. Where licensing is deemed necessary, we recommend a national licensing law, which would allow for increased labor mobility.

2. We recommend that the federal government help finance the training of the newer health occupations, such as physician's assistants. There is little likelihood that in the near future this nation will train or acquire a sufficient number of physicians to meet its health care needs.

3. We recommend the establishment of a national performance review to oversee the rate setting policies of hospitals. At The Cambridge Hospital, approximately 75 percent of the hospital bills are paid by third-party payers (a substantial increase over two years ago). During the same period, the hospital's losses have

decreased from approximately $1.5 million (1968) to $.8 million (1970).

4. Few doctors are attracted into the practice of family or general medicine. Because of greater earning opportunities as specialists and because some stigma is attached to being a general practitioner, the vast majority of medical students specialize. We recommend that the federal government increase the number of physicians at the primary entry points by financially encouraging medical schools to train "people doctors" (or family physicians) who would combine the appropriate specialties. These federally financed grants, made either directly to medical students or to medical schools, should be conditional. The principal condition should be two or four years of public service employment after graduation in areas of the nation experiencing the greatest shortages of physicians, for example, rural communities and urban ghettos.

5. We recommend that the federal government financially support the hiring of hospital consultants who have expertise in implementing new occupational patterns. Hospital administrators generally do not have much knowledge of this special area of manpower utilization.

6. We recommend that commissioners of health, chiefs of medicine, and hospital adiministrators carefully study these recommendations to determine the feasibility of implementing some or all of them in their own hospitals.

7. Since there is a relative shortage of RNs and LPNs, we recommend that these two occupations be eased out of low-level functions in general nursing; these functions should be performed by persons in occupations requiring less education and training.

8. Since the traditional occupational hierarchy prohibits vertical mobility, we recommend that hospitals juxtapose an alternative that permits upward mobility through in-service training and education. Such alternatives could include the establishment of new paramedical occupations, such as nursing assistant, medical assistant, and physician's assistant.

9. Hospitals should reexamine their paramedical occupational structures to determine realistic job requirements for each occupation.

10. Hospitals should establish hiring-in standards that are relevant to the functions to be performed by each occupation. Arbitrary licensing and unnecessary education requirements should be eliminated.

11. Hospitals should expand their in-service training programs for selected paramedical employees where it is clear that these employees can be trained for better-paying positions. For paramedical occupations, in-service training is likely to be more efficient and economical.

12. Hospitals should improve their in-service education programs for paramedical and medical workers, thereby permitting them to keep abreast of the constantly changing techniques and technology.

13. In many instances hospitals find themselves insufficiently financed or too small to assume the financial burden of in-service training and education. In these cases, we recommend that hospitals provide in-service training and education through arrangements with neighboring hospitals and educational institutions on a cooperative basis.

4

The Five Hospital Study: Objectives and Methodology

The principal objectives of the *Five Hospital Study,* which began in 1973, was to test the findings of The Cambridge Hospital study in a number of different settings. Was the situation in The Cambridge Hospital unique because of factors such as its administrators, its size, or its status as a municipal hospital? Would the findings be repeated in a variety of hospitals facing different sets of circumstances? The basic hypothesis to be tested was that the findings of the study in The Cambridge Hospital would be confirmed in a small but diverse sample of hospitals. The assumption was that if the hypothesis were confirmed, the findings would encourage many hospitals across the nation to analyze their occupational structures and to apply the restructuring techniques and policies that were successful in The Cambridge Hospital.

The methodology for the *Five Hospital Study* was a product of our experiences in the two previous projects, *Hiring Standards for Paramedical Manpower* (HSPM) and *Restructuring of Paramedical Occupations* (RPO). The plan incorporated the list of functions compiled by the HSPM study; these were cross-checked with interviews conducted in the initial phase of The Cambridge Hospital (RPO) study, and the interview form was then refined further. The final version was put in the same form as the functional questionnaries used in the RPO study. Both the number of health occupations and of the detailed functional questions within each occupations were substantially increased over the numbers in our previous studies.

One of the principal goals of the research was to determine the amount of overlap in the performance of medical functions by occupational categories, each category representing a varying level of education, training, and experience. To accomplish this, the questionnaires were designed so that associated occupational categories would be able to respond to the same questions. The following is a list of occupations for which questionnaires were developed and the nine categories to which they are applicable:

1. *General nursing service:*
   Registered nurse
   Licensed practical nurse
   Nurse's aide
   Orderly
   Nursing assistant
   Senior nursing assistant
   Nursing technician
   Senior nursing technician
2. *Primary care:*
   Physician
     Intern
     Resident
   Nurse practitioners
   Pediatric nurse practitioner
   Physician's assistant
   Registered nurse
3. *Laboratory:*
   Hematology technician
   Hematology technologist
   Blood bank technician
   Blood bank technologist
   Bacteriology technician
   Bacteriology technologist
   Cytology technician
   Cytology technologist
   Histology technician
   Histology technologist

Urinalysis and parasitology
  technician
Urinalysis and parasitology
  technologist
Chemistry technician
Chemistry technologist
4. *Operating room:*
   Registered nurse
   Licensed practical nurse
   Surgical technician
   Operating room orderly
5. *Inhalation therapy:*
   Inhalation technologist
   Inhalation technician
6. *Radiology:*
   Radiology technologist
   Radiology technician
7. *EKG:*
   EKG technician
8. *Psychiatry:*
   Registered nurse
   Psychiatric attendant
9. *Clerical:*
   Ward secretary
   Unit clerk
   Unit secretary
   Unit aide

The basic methodology used in *The Cambridge Hospital Study* (summarized in chapter 3) was applied to the five cooperating hospitals. The hospitals were selected to represent a mix of facility size, locations, services, and staffing requirements.

The five cooperating hospitals are described in detail in chapter 5, but the following is a brief description of each (fictitious names are used to avoid indentification):

1. Adonis is a 500-bed, short-term, municipal, teaching hospital serving low income residents of the inner city. Only its pediatrics department was included in the study.

2. Bacchus is a short-term, private, general, nonprofit teaching hospital with 300 beds serving an upper and middle income urban population.

3. Cressyda is a large, short-term, private, nonprofit hospital with 322 beds serving a rural population with mixed incomes.

4. Desdemona is a private, short-term, nonprofit hospital with 75 beds serving a low income urban population.

5. Elektra is a short-term, municipal, teaching hospital with 200 beds, serving a low and lower-middle income urban population.

Personal interviews were conducted with a sample of health workers in the nineteen occupations included in this study. The interviews consisted of two parts, a general background questionnaire for all respondents, followed by the functions questionnaire for the appropriate occupational category. A total of 275 interviews was completed. Table 11 gives the number of employees interviewed in each category and in each hospital.

As table 11 shows, about three-quarters of the interviews were equally divided among three facilities, Adonis (pediatrics), Bacchus, and Elektra. The remaining quarter was divided between Cressyda, where the interviews were conducted only within the nursing department, and Desdemona, which is a relatively small facility.

The breakdown of the total by occupation reflects the concentration of our efforts in the nursing department: 53.3 percent of all the interviews were in the registered nurse, licensed practical nurse, or nurse's aide categories. Laboratory personnel accounted for 10.2 percent of the sample; x-ray technicians, 6.3 percent; and inhalation therapists, 4.7 percent. Physicians were included in the study for the first time and represented 3.5 percent

Table 11. The Number of Personnel Interviewed by Hospital and Occupational Category

Occupation	Adonis (pediatrics only)	Bacchus Hospital	Cressyda Hospital	Desdemona Hospital	Elektra Hospital	Total	Percent distribution of occupations interviewed
Physician	9	—	—	—	—	9	3.5
Nurse practitioner	—	—	—	—	2	2	.8
Pediatric nurse practitioner	—	—	—	—	4	4	1.6
Registered nurse	22	15	5	7	12	61	23.7
Licensed practical nurse	3	4	3	4	3	17	6.6
Nurse's aide	16	6	24	7	6	59	23.0
Surgical nurse	—	2	—	1	1	4	1.6
Surgical technician	—	2	—	1	2	5	1.9
Surgical aide	—	1	—	—	1	2	.8
Laboratory technician	2	11	—	4	9	26	10.1
X-ray technician	2	8	—	2	4	16	6.2
Inhalation therapy technician	—	6	—	3	3	12	4.7
EKG technician	—	1	—	1	1	3	1.2
Psychiatric nurse	—	—	—	—	2	2	.8
Psychiatric attendant	—	—	—	—	1	1	.4
Neighborhood health worker	—	—	—	—	2	2	.8
Ward secretary	6	9	—	4	2	21	8.2
Unit aide	—	2	—	—	2	2	.8
Medical records personnel	—	4	—	1	4	9	3.5
Total	60	71	32	35	59	257	100.2
Percent distribution of interviews by hospital	23.3	27.6	12.4	13.3	23.0	99.9	

Source: CMMS Survey

of the total interviewed. Other than the ward secretary group, which represented 8.2 percent, the remaining interviews were distributed principally among technicians and surgical occupations.

It should be noted that the number interviewed as a percentage of total employees in a category varied widely between facilities and occupations. The sample was chosen at random, and the minumum was a 15 percent sample in those occupations with a large number of employees. However, in occupations employing only one or two persons, the sample was 50 or 100 percent. In order not to mislead the reader, the total number interviewed has been included at the bottom of each table. For example, the report of 50 percent of a sample of fourteen on the performance of a certain function may be more reliable than the report of 50 percent of a sample of two.

Sixty interviews covering six occupations were conducted in the pediatrics department of Adonis Hospital. The pediatrics department relies on the adult department for most technical services, so laboratory, x-ray, and other technical employment is limited. The number of registered nurses interviewed represented a majority of those employed. These interviews provided the first opportunity to use the patient care questionnaire with nursing personnel. This questionnaire was an extensive, itemized list of functions combining all general nursing functions with the more complex functions usually assigned to physicians.

The general nursing functions from the patient care questionnaire were also analyzed separately for each occupational group to which the questionnaire was administered. This allowed comparison of different workers — from nurse's aide to physician — who at times perform the same functions. All the interviews conducted at Cressyda were in the nursing department because of its extensive in-service training program for nurse's aides (see chapter 5). As noted on table 11, there were twenty-four nurse's aides interviewed from that hospital. The breakdown of respondents from the in-service program was eight nursing asssistants, three senior nursing assistants, eight nursing technicians, and five senior nursing technicians. The registered nurses and licensed practical nurses were interviewed to determine how the in-service program affected their duties.

Nurse practitioners, registered nurses, and the house staff at Adonis were included to assess the overlap in the performance of "marginal medical" functions by physicians, nurse practitioners, and registered nurses. (The nurse practitioners are employed at neighborhood health centers affiliated with Elektra Hospital.)

When each questionnaire had been tallied, we compiled tables that show the average percent of time spent per function as well as the average percent of workers in each category who perform each function. With this information it is possible to make comparisons between occupations to determine the amount of overlap that exists.

The responses for all but the general nursing data were calculated by using the average percent of time spent by each occupation on each function. In addition, the ratio of performers to the total number interviewed was expressed in percentage terms. From this information it was possible to determine the average amount of time spent on each function as well as the number of those interviewed who performed each function. These two statistics provide the information necessary to discover how extensive the overlap is and which occupations are affected.

A summary table (similar to table 6) was developed to show the distribution of time spent by nursing occupations within the nursing department on functions grouped by level of difficulty. The following is a breakdown of these levels of difficulty:

Level	Functions	
I	1-18	Simplest
II	19-30	More difficult
III	31-47	Most difficult
IV	48-63	Supervisory functions
V	64-69	Pediatric functions

In making comparisons, emphasis should be placed on levels I, II, and III, which are differentiated strictly according to the difficulty of functions.

The following is a detailed, step-by-step outline of the method used to construct the summary table. This method overcomes the problems associated with a summary by eliminating the effect of the variation in the number of performers for each function.

1. Evaluate each questionnaire and reduce the percentage of time spent on each function proportionately so that the total equals 100. To accomplish this — following the instructions on the questionnaire — total the percentage of time spent on all functions and divide 100 by this total. The result is a reducing factor that will decrease the given percents to actual percentage, totaling 100.

2. Using the worksheet (sample appended to chapter 8), transfer the actual percentage of time spent on each function for all interviewed in an occupation. (We have entered Susan Jones's interview results in the column headed "Interview I" on the sample page.)

3. Add across the row for the percent of time spent by individuals 1, 2, 3, and 4 on each function and enter totals in column A.

4. Multiply each entry in column A by 2,400 (minutes in an average work week) and enter in column B to get the total minutes spent on each function by those who perform it.

5. Add the total minutes spent on each group of functions in column B and enter these group totals in the box provided on the worksheet.

6. Calculate the percentage of time spent on each group by dividing each group total by the grand total and entering it in the column labeled "% by Group." These percentage figures are the summary table breakdown for each occupation.

The Interviews

Interviews were conducted away from the work situation to avoid distraction. The interviewer asked the questions orally and recorded all the responses. This method was adopted for several reasons: first, this allowed for further explanation if required; second, the respondent could focus on one question at a time; third, use of a single interviewer minimized personal bias in recording answers and percentages.

Each session was prefaced by a brief explanation of the project. In addition, the interviewer assured each respondent that the interview was confidential and that no names would be associated with individual responses. The first part of the interview consisted of background information in which previous education and training, as well as work experience, were recorded. Further questions focused on the orientation received for the present job. This was then compared to what the respondents felt should have been their orientation. The next questions were addressed to the respondents' perception of their work, their satisfaction with the occupation and the employer, and their view of the possibilities for advancement. Since much of this information consisted of private evaluations that might have influenced future work relationships, especially with supervisors, the stipulation that the responses were confidential was essential to collect meaningful data.

The second part of the interview consisted of a list of functions that represented tasks performed within these occupations. As we noted earlier, the basic questionnaires were developed during two previous projects, *Hiring Standards for Paramedical Manpower* and *Restructuring Paramedical Occupations,* but substantial additions were made for this study.

The respondents were asked to estimate how much of their time was spent on each function. The following is a guideline that was used to help them in estimating their time.

Based on a 40-hour workweek:

If a performer spends:	*It is recorded in percent:*
Under 20 minutes	less than 1 percent
30 minutes-2 hours	1-5 percent
2 hours-4 hours	6-10 percent
4 hours-6 hours	11-15 percent
6 hours-10 hours	16-25 percent
over 10 hours	greater than 25 percent

The respondents were permitted to use either time (in minutes or hours) or percentages, but the final distribution in this study is described in percentages. The underlying assumption is that while there is little response bias in the way respondents break down their time, there may be inconsistency in the numbers they choose to use. Therefore, if the total percentage of time spent on the functions did not equal 100 percent, each function was weighted for the final tabulation so that the total did equal 100 percent.

The general outline of the interview procedures, the guidelines for evaluating the results, and the techniques used to tabulate them have been included for two reasons. We want to present the method used to obtain our results, and we want to provide a model for others who may wish to use this approach in some other facility.

A sample interview, representing typical responses from a registered nurse, is appended to chapter 8. The answers are then included as interview 1 in the sample worksheet that follows the interview.

5

Profiles of the Five Hospitals

As indicated earlier, fictitious names were used for the five hospitals, in order to hide their identity. The following is a description of each hospital studied. The statistics are summarized in tables 12 and 13.

Adonis

Adonis Hospital opened in the late 1800s. It is a short-term, general, municipal hospital. As a teaching hospital, it was affiliated with three medical schools until the early 1970s, when it restructured its affiliations and became associated with only one. In 1977 the hospital had more than four hundred and fifty beds and a staffing complement of over three thousand.

Adonis has been a pioneer in the development of radiology, pathology research, and clinical investigation. In conjunction with its extensive facilities for patient care, it conducts full university training for physicians, both undergraduate and postgraduate. All departments are professionally affiliated with a university medical center, a modern medical complex immediately adjacent to the hospital.

The medical center clinical complex contains complete inpatient and outpatient facilities in surgery, medicine, pediatrics, ob-

Table 12. Comparison of Selected Utilization Statistics for the Five Hospitals, 1972-75

Hospitals	Beds		Admissions		Average daily census		Occupancy rate (in percent)		Expenses (in thousands) Total		Payroll		Other		Personnel	
	1972	1975	1972	1975	1972	1975	1972	1975	1972	1975	1972	1975	1972	1975	1972	1975
Adonis[1]	809	500	21812	16765	630	393	76.0	78.6	45629	55130	31372	35409	14257	19721	3669	2988
Bacchus	309	300	8886	8796	227	232	73.5	77.3	13097	16432	7463	9075	5634	7357	605	985
Cressyda	322	317	9580	10160	235	240	73.0	73.2	7870	10322	4451	4915	3419	5407	753	844
Desdemona	75	75	2085	1962	58	52	77.3	69.3	2400	2966	1436	1613	964	1293	172	188
Elektra	187	185	6865	7159	141	157	75.4	84.0	8023	11635	4803	6421	3220	5214	647	628

Source: *Hospital Statistics*, American Hospital Association, 1973, 1976 editions.

[1]These figures are for the entire hospital, including pediatrics.

Table 13. Percentage Change in Selected Utilization Statistics for the Five Hospitals, 1972-75

Hospitals	Beds	Admissions	Average daily census	Occupancy rate (percent)	Expenses			Personnel
					Total	Payroll	Other	
Adonis[1]								
Bacchus	-2.9	-1.0	2.2	5.2	25.5	21.6	30.6	62.8
Cressyda	-1.6	6.1	2.1	.3	31.2	10.4	58.1	12.1
Desdemona	—	-5.9	-10.3	-10.3	21.2	12.3	34.1	4.7
Elektra	-1.1	4.3	11.3	11.4	45.0	33.7	61.9	-2.9

Source: Calculated from data on table 12.

[1]Figures for pediatrics alone were not available.

stetrics, and psychiatry. One of the nation's busiest emergency services is located at Adonis, with approximately 130,000 visits per year; the hospital provides about 133,000 days of patient care annually and has almost 15,800 discharges.

The Northeastern University Center for Medical Manpower Studies was involved only with the pediatrics department of Adonis and its satellite neighborhood health centers, whose major focus is delivering services to children. Pediatrics admits about three thousand children a year and more than seventy thousand are seen in ambulatory services. Approximately two thousand infants are delivered by the obstetrical service each year. In addition to routine outpatient care, an active pediatrics emergency accident floor operates around the clock. Much effort has been devoted to developing a primary care pathway so the delivery of care will be a continous experience for patients both within the hospital and in neighborhood health centers.

Bacchus

Bacchus Hospital is a 300-bed, short-term, general, not-for-profit, community hospital founded in the late 1800s. The hospital is now affiliated with three medical schools. It runs its own nursing school and is associated with two college nursing programs as well. There are other allied health education programs within the hospital, notably a training program for radiology technicians.

This hospital provides both inpatient and outpatient services for a population area of about three hundred thousand persons. Services include departments of medicine, surgery, psychiatry, obstetrics, pediatrics, round the clock ambulatory care, and an evening clinic for young people.

Recently, three new buildings were completed, including an ambulatory care center that combines emergency with nonemergency care. The outpatient facility handled almost sixty-five thousand visits in 1973, an increase of nearly 46 percent over the 1968 figure.

The revitalization of the emergency area focused on a new system of staffing and organization that made services more accessible and improved the quality of care. The number of people seeking outpatient treatment at Bacchus jumped by 190 percent during the years 1974-76.

In an innovative approach to outpatient care, the staffing arrangement of the outpatient department ensures that patients receive continuity of care, a factor that had previously been ignored. A new referral system has been developed so in the initial visit, the patient's medical needs are assessed and he or she is given the names of private physicians whose location, specialty, and other characteristics are matched to the patient's needs. The patient also has the option of returning to the outpatient department, in which case Bacchus acts as the primary physician. A sliding fee scale, based on professional time and the level of service, has been established so that even the uninsured can afford care.

Between 1972 and 1975, the number of beds declined by 2.9 percent, the occupancy rate increased by 5.2 percent, the number of admissions fell slightly (1 percent), while the average daily census increased by 2.2 percent. Total expenses during this period increased by 25.5 percent, payroll expenses increased by 21.6 percent, and all others by 30.6 percent. In 1972 payroll expenses accounted for 57 percent of all expenses and in 1975, 55.2 percent. This occurred while the total number of employees increased by 62.8 percent.

Cressyda

Cressyda is a private, short-term, nonprofit facility located in a northern New England city with a population of thirty thousand persons. The area is mostly rural and there is a shortage of physicians in general practice. The hospital, in cooperation with eighteen community hospitals, serves as the principal source of health care for the entire region. It provides a wide range of services, including intensive care and cardiac intensive care units, diagnostic and therapeutic radioisotope facilities, physical therapy, inhalation therapy, well-organized outpatient and emergency departments, and a long-term care unit.

The medical center has an extensive enrollment in its nationally accredited school of nursing, nurse anesthesia, medical laboratory, technology, and radiography programs. In addition, there are certificate programs in coronary care nursing and intravenous therapy. Because of shorter periods of hospitalization, a program of discharge education has been developed to help train the patient in proper self-care at home.

Steps have been taken during the past five years to respond to the changing health needs of the community. A major innovation has been the development of a broadly based outpatient/emergency department. The number of visits to this department has risen markedly as it has become known for its emphasis on a "family screening process." The unit is staffed by physicians twenty-four hours a day and provides access or referrals to diagnostic and treatment services.

The Center for Medical Manpower Studies became involved with the hospital when it opened a six-story patient tower and expanded its auxiliary care facilities with a major ambulatory care center. The total bed complement remained about the same. However, the principal emphasis for the entire project was on the expansion and modernization of ancillary and outpatient service areas rather than on inpatient growth.

From 1972 to 1975, the number of beds declined 1.6 percent, the number of admissions increased 6.1 percent, the average daily census increased 2.1 percent, while the occupancy rate remained about the same. In 1972, the number of emergency/outpatient visits had increased by more than two and a half times the 1969 level. In 1972, there were nearly twenty-six thousand visits reported.

Among the five hospitals studied, Cressyda experienced the second greatest increase in costs over the three-year period 1972-1975, a sizable 31.2 percent. More than 80 percent of the increase may be attributed to expenses other than payroll. In spite of an increase of 12.1 percent in the number of employees, the hospital was able to control its payroll expenses so that it experienced the smallest increase in payroll of the five hospitals studied, 10.4 percent.

The success in limiting personnel costs is the result of an extensive in-service training program that provides a supply of well-trained personnel at a signifcantly reduced cost.

Cressyda Hospital has an in-service training program providing upgrading opportunities for its allied health personnel. There are five stages to this program within the nursing department: (1) nursing assistant, (2) senior nursing assistant, (3) nursing technician, (4) senior nursing technician, and (5) LPN by waiver. In addition, there is a "co-op" training program for area high school students.

If the new employees (male or female) have no previous training in this field, they become nursing assistant trainees. A high school diploma is not required for this position. This program is a five-week course consisting of about half formal classes and half on-the-job training. First, a nursing assistant trainee is assigned to a nursing technician who is responsible throughout the training program for teaching new procedures and techniques. The trainee is given a procedure check list, which is signed by a nursing technician or head nurse when a procedure is satisfactorily performed. This chart is kept available on the ward so that newly mastered tasks can be checked off daily. When this chart is complete, it is placed in the trainee's employment record in the nursing service office.

The trainee is assigned to a medical ward for a two-week period and then a surgical ward for another two-week training period. The final week of training is spent in the ward to which the trainee will be permanently assigned. This period also includes classroom teaching one day a week so that the in-service supervisor may review procedures previously taught, as well as give demonstrations of and nursing conferences on new procedures and techniques. After the third week, the trainee may be assigned an individual patient with the approval of the head nurse and the in-service supervisor. The trainee has the same schedule and assignment as the nursing technician, and the latter is responsible for teaching and reviewing new procedures as well as for supervision of nursing care during the five-week period. At the end of the fifth week, the nursing technician gives a complete review of the implementation of nursing procedures on the ward. The trainee is then evaluated by the head nurse, by the nursing technician who has been assigned to the trainee, and by the in-service supervisor.

The course is offered according to need, when both the number of available positions and the number of interested applicants warrant it. Advancement beyond the entry-level position is made on the basis of demonstrated proficiency, usually at the end of a year of employment. The amount of time needed to become a senior nursing assistant varies with the individual and has been as short as six months.

A nursing technician may elect to take the state board examination to become a waiver licensed practical nurse. A waiver LPN may perform all the functions of an LPN except to give medications and be the charge person. However, if a nursing technician chooses to enter a formal LPN program, no advance credit is given for the on-the-job training received at the hospital.

The entire list of salary scales and advancements within the nursing department as of January 1973 is listed below:

Occupation	Weekly Salary Ranges
Nursing assistant trainee:	$ 72.00 - $ 80.00
Senior nursing assistant:	78.40 - 86.90
Nursing technician:	85.20 - 94.80
Senior nursing technician:	88.80 - 98.40
Waiver LPN:	88.80 - 98.40
LPN:	95.50 - 106.50
Registered nurse (general duty):	140.00 - 155.00

In addition to this highly developed in-service training program, Cressyda also offers extensive continuing education, and review classes are scheduled whenever there is a change in hospital policy or procedure. In addition, there are optional nursing classes available to the entire nursing staff — for example, a cardiac care course and EKG training.

LPNs at Cressyda are accepted as skilled enough to work in the intensive care unit (ICU) and the cardiac care unit (CCU). LPNs are also encouraged to attend the coronary care course.

The nursing assistants and technicians who participate in the in-service training program are highly regarded and also thought to be competent enough to work in the ICU and CCU. Table 14

shows the distribution of the nursing assistant and nursing
technician staff at the time the interviews were conducted (1973).

Table 14. Distribution of Assistant and Nursing Technician Staff at
         Cressyda Hospital, 1973

Staff	Number full time	Number part time	Total	Percent distribution*
Nursing assistant	24	3	27	23.3
Senior nursing assistant	23	6	29	25.0
Nursing technician	35	16	51	44.0
Senior nursing technician	7	2	9	7.8
Total	89	27	116	100.1

*Totals may not add to 100.0 percent because of rounding.

Desdemona

Desdemona Hospital was founded in the late 1800s as a sixteen-
bed facility. It is now a private, short-term, nonprofit, general
hospital with seventy-five beds located in a small city within a
metropolitian area. The city has undergone a number of changes
in recent years, in particular a steady loss of population overall,
accompanied by a significant increase within the black and
Spanish-speaking communities. The hospital provides blood
bank, inhalation therapy, physical therapy, and diagnostic radioisotope services. In addition, there are organized outpatient and
emergency services which have been expanded to meet changing
community needs.

The hospital recently expanded its services to include
comprehensive emergency room care twenty-four hours a day.
Care is provided in an informal program that is coordinated with a
health center located on the hospital grounds and a number of
other health providers located in the community.

Since 1972 when the Center for Medical Manpower Studies
became involved with the hospital, certain changes in utilization
patterns have occurred. Although the number of beds remained
constant, the number of admissions declined by 5.9 percent, the
average daily census dropped from fifty-eight to fifty-two, and the

occupancy rate fell by 8 percent. These changes reflect the hospital's current emphasis on expansion of outpatient services, which in turn is a reflection of changing community needs. Personnel increased by 4 percent, but the proportion of labor costs in the total costs declined. Labor accounted for 59.8 percent of total costs in 1972, but only 55.5 percent in 1975.

Elektra

Elektra is a short-term, municipal, general, teaching hospital located in a medium-sized city with a large number of low income families. It offers a number of services, including physical therapy, laboratory services, extensive inpatient and outpatient psychiatric care, and emergency and outpatient facilities.

It was established in 1917 under a state charter to provide for the "sick poor" of the city. The small three-story building contained 50 beds. It was owned, operated, and financed by the city and was staffed by civil service employees. In 1946 two wings were added to house a school of nursing and a 100-bed maternity building. At that time, the main building housed about two hundred and fifty patients in large open wards.

As early as 1960 it was evident that the facilities were either deteriorating or becoming obsolete. The hospital continued to run at a deficit. It became more difficult to recruit a competent house staff and the overall reputation of the hospital was poor. During the period 1963-66, change occurred rapidly. A medical school agreed to an affiliation and the hospital was no longer dependent on foreign-trained physicians for its house staff. In addition, the financial picture improved. One of the old buildings was razed, and work on a $10 million facility was begun.

The impact of these changes was far-reaching. Many employees who had worked for many years at the hospital with little change in their duties reacted with fear and suspicion to the new environment. Community physicians were also wary of the changes. The affiliated university appointed chiefs of services and filled the hospital with bright, energetic residents. New policies were created, new procedures instituted, and new systems implemented. Throughout this transition period, there was evidence of strain in many areas.

From 1972 to 1975 the number of beds in Elektra declined from 187 to 185. However, there were significant increases in the number of admissions (4.3 percent), average daily census (11.3 percent), and occupancy rate, which increased by 8.6 percentage points (from 75.4 in 1972 to 84 percent in 1975).

During this period Elektra experienced the largest increase in total expenses of any of the five hospitals studied, a substantial 45 percent. Nearly half of this increase was the result of increases in payroll while nonlabor costs accounted for the rest. Payroll expenses increased by 33.7 percent while the remaining expenses increased by 61.9 percent. Municipal workers also negotiated for and received significant increases in wages, which strained the hospital budget, but there was a decline of only 2.9 percent in hospital employees during this period.

6

Analysis of Data on Medical Functions

The discussion and analysis presented below is based on 257 separate formal interviews with hospital personnel. The interviews were completed in the hospitals by our own research staff over the period of the project. In addition, hundreds of informal interviews and discussions took place during the research period. A broad range of health occupations was studied, and our investigation produced nearly three hundred pages of statistical tables.[1] All these data and reports were synthesized and summarized, and the following is an analysis of the data on medical functions.

General Nursing

Of the 257 documented interviews, 145 — or 56 percent — were in the general nursing category. General nursing usually represents one of the largest employment areas for any health provider. Of these 145 interviews conducted in general nursing, 9 were with physicians, 60 with RNs, 17 with LPNs, and 59 with nurse's aides.

Although physicians would not generally consider themselves part of general nursing, we included them for a specific reason: physicians spend significant amounts of time performing medical tasks that are also performed by less highly trained health care personnel. Perhaps the last statement should be reversed. Over the last five decades allied health occupations have increasingly taken over functions traditionally performed only by the physicians. Health providers have become more and more aware of this phenomenon. The pertinent questions at this point are: How far has this trend progressed, and what, if anything, should be the reaction of health providers?

Table 15 provides a summary view of four categories of personnel who provide nursing care in the five hospitals. As described in the chapter on methodology, the medical care functions have been grouped into five categories. Groups I, II, and III are ranked in order of difficulty, from easiest to most difficult. Group IV functions are administrative in nature and group V functions are related to care of the newborn only, so comparisons based on difficulty of the tasks will be most fruitful in groups I, II, and III.

The date in table 15 indicate that 49.6 percent of the nine MDs spend 23.4 percent of their time on group I functions, while 76.7 percent of the sixty RNs spend 27.7 percent of their time on the same relatively easy functions. Of the seventeen LPNs, 82.7 percent spend 26.1 percent of their time on these functions, and 81.1 percent of the fifty-nine NAs spend 57.2 percent of their time on them.

Looking at group III functions, we see that 69.7 percent of the MDs spend 26.6 percent of their time on these tasks, 70.6 percent of the RNs spend 24.5 percent of their time, 64.7 percent of the LPNs spend 20.8 percent of their time, and 34.1 percent of the NAs spend 8.1 percent of their time on the most difficult set of medical functions.

The data on table 15 indicate that persons with sophisticated training and formal education (MDs and RNs) tend to spend greater amounts of time on the most difficult medical functions; conversely, less time is spent on these functions by less highly trained and less formally educated personnel. However, it is also noteworthy that some members of each occupational category spend at least part of their time performing tasks at each level of difficulty.

Table 15. Average Percent of Performers (1) and Average Percent of Performers' Total Time (2) Spent on Five Groups of Functions at Five Hospitals by Physicians, Registered Nurses, Licensed Practical Nurses, and Nurse's Aides

Groups of functions ranked from easiest to most difficult	MDs (1)	MDs (2)	RNs (1)	RNs (2)	LPNs (1)	LPNs (2)	NAs (1)	NAs (2)
Group I (1-18)	49.6	23.4	76.7	27.7	82.7	26.1	81.8	57.2
Group II (19-30)	44.4	10.7	82.4	23.7	80.9	31.3	68.8	29.0
Group III (31-47)	69.7	26.6	70.6	24.5	64.7	20.8	34.1	8.1
Group IV (48-63)	65.0	39.1	71.7	21.1	48.5	15.5	20.0	10.2
Group V (64-69)	na	ná	11.4	3.1	13.7	7.5	7.8	1.5
Number of performers	9		60		17		59	

Source: H.M. Goldstein and M.A. Horowitz, *Utilization of Health Personnel: A Five Hospital Study*, Vol. 2. (Appendix). A Report to the U.S. Department of Labor, Employment and Training Administration, March 1978. Calculated from table A-2, appendix, pp. A9–A17.

Physicians spend a portion of their time on easy functions, and a sizable percentage of NAs, despite their minimum training and formal education, spend considerable amounts of time on the most sophisticated medical functions listed. Table 15 also shows that more persons with higher levels of formal education and medical training spend more time on administrative functions than those with less formal education and training. However, all personnel, regardless of training, do at times perform administrative tasks.

A study of table 16, which describes data for individual hospitals, indicates few major deviations from the aggregate figures shown in table 15. At Cressyda relatively more of the NAs (93 percent) spend slightly more than average amounts of time on the easiest functions. At the same time relatively more LPNs (83.2 percent) spend slightly more than average amounts of time on group III functions, and a significantly higher percentage of NAs (54.6 percent compared to an average of 34.1 percent) spend time on group III functions.

The relatively efficient use of health manpower at Cressyda Hospital must in some measure be credited to its well-organized in-service training program which provides realistic upgrading opportunities for employees. (A description of the hospital's training activities is outlined in chapter 5.)

In addition to our general nursing questionnnaire, which ranked 69 medical tasks by order of difficulty, we developed a more extensive patient care questionnaire. This listed 279 marginal medical functions, including the 69 general nursing tasks from the nursing questionnaire. The more extensive patient care questionnaire was used only at Adonis Hospital because this was the only institution where physicians were included in our sample. Nine physicians, two nurse practitioners, and three pediatric nurse practitioners, as well as twenty-two registered nurses, were asked to respond to the extended questionnaire. The list of functions comprised general duties such as "doing errands for patients" or "straightening up and cleaning patients' rooms"; technical tasks such as "operating EKG equipment" or "identifying abnormal cardiac rhythms on EKG"; and emergency procedures such as "intubating trachea" or "performing a cardiac massage."

Table 16. Average Percent of Performers (1) and Average Percent of Time (2) Spent on Five Groups of Functions at Each of Five Hospitals by Registered Nurses, Licensed Practical Nurses, and Nurse's Aides.

Groups of functions ranked from easiest to most difficult	RN (1)	RN (2)	LPN (1)	LPN (2)	NA (1)	NA (2)
Group I (1-18)						
Hospital Adonis	75.0	25.3	74.0	20.5	63.9	54.7
Hospital Bacchus	74.6	26.0	73.6	30.5	80.6	51.8
Hospital Cressyda	80.0	20.5	90.0	31.1	93.0	45.7
Hospital Desdemona	71.4	25.6	86.1	44.1	77.7	48.5
Hospital Elektra	87.5	34.3	87.0	21.3	84.2	49.1
Group II (14-30)						
Hospital A	84.5	25.6	88.9	32.1	44.8	26.8
Hospital B	80.0	21.1	89.5	37.0	75.0	32.1
Hospital C	84.0	16.0	86.6	29.7	74.2	33.8
Hospital D	75.0	26.0	87.5	30.8	75.0	36.9
Hospital E	83.3	21.8	75.0	21.6	65.2	27.8
Group III (31-47)						
Hospital A	79.2	25.7	50.0	19.7	24.2	14.9
Hospital B	83.0	22.6	76.8	20.8	27.0	8.2
Hospital C	86.0	25.2	83.2	22.1	54.6	11.8
Hospital D	71.4	39.4	59.3	14.1	33.9	10.4
Hospital E	75.5	23.2	70.8	20.8	40.6	9.3
Group IV (48-63) (Admin.)						
Hospital A	74.6	23.3	62.5	25.7	5.0	2.5
Hospital B	69.6	20.1	34.3	10.6	4.1	5.8
Hospital C	88.0	38.3	80.0	16.1	31.3	7.8
Hospital D	32.1	7.6	39.0	9.6	11.6	3.0
Hospital E	76.5	18.0	54.1	8.4	26.0	8.0
Group V (64-69) (Newborn)						
Hospital A	1.8	.1	1.8	2.0	7.5	1.0
Hospital B	30.9	10.1	12.5	1.0	16.6	2.1
Hospital C	20.0	.1	66.6	.9	4.2	.8
Hospital D	7.1	1.3	12.5	1.4	11.4	1.0
Hospital E	12.5	2.1	22.2	27.9	20.0	5.7

Source: *Utilization of Health Personnel: A Five Hospital Study,* Vol. 2, Calculated from background data, appendix.

Table 17 shows eight functions chosen arbitrarily from the questionnaire and the extent to which personnel from each category perform each of the functions. The amount of time spent on a particular function and the type of professional performing it does not appear to follow a rational pattern. In fact, more than 80 percent of the 279 patient care functions were performed at some time by members of all four categories. Table 18 displays the overlap of responsibility for all 279 functions. Like much of the other data generated by our investigation, the responses to the patient care questionnaire suggest that hospital tasks are performed by the medical personnel who happen to be available, with little regard for the training, certification, or degree of competence of the individuals involved.

Nursing Personnel

In this section on nursing personnel, three separate units are analyzed: operating room, emergency room, and outpatient department.

Operating Room

Of the 275 formal interviews, 11 (or 4.3 percent) were with operating room personnel, who were employed at three of the five hospitals.[2] Of these 11 interviews, 4 were with RNs, 5 were with technicians, and 2 were with NAs. An examination of the functional questionnaires for operating room personnel indicates that most functions, irrespective of the degree of difficulty, were performed by both RNs and technicians. The NAs performed fewer functions, but the ones they did perform were scattered between the "easy" and "difficult" levels. There does not seem to be any relationship between the formal educational qualifications of individuals and the type of task they performed in the operating room. The distribution of time by those who performed the operating room functions is similar across categories—that is, usually when an RN spends a certain percentage of time on a function, whether "easy" or "difficult," a similar proportion of time will be spent on the same function by the less formally trained technician. At several of the hospitals, operating room technicians were trained on the job. They originally were what would normally be considered entry-level personnel.

Emergency Room

Of the 275 interviews, 11 (or 4.3 percent) were with emergency room personnel.[3] Of these eleven performers, seven were RNs, four were NAs, and all were employed in three of the five hospitals. Eight of the eleven were employed at Adonis Hospital (four RNs and four NAs). RNs at Adonis Hospital performed fifty-four of the sixty-nine medical functions (78 percent). NAs at this same institution performed thirty-eight of the sixty-nine medical functions (55 percent). There is an indication that as the functions became more difficult, fewer of the NAs were involved. However, the trend is not very strong. Many of the NAs performed the more complex emergency room functions and spend significant amounts of time on them. Equally important is the finding that RNs in the emergency room allotted substantial amounts of time to the relatively simple functions.

Outpatient Department

Seven of the persons interviewed (2.7 percent) were assigned to the outpatient departments in three of the five hospitals.[4] Adonis Hospital employed four of these seven (two RNs and two NAs). All four performed the majority of the sixty-nine functions, and the proportion of time spent on these functions does not appear to be related to licensure, certification, or formal professional training. RNs performed most of the easy, as well as most of the difficult, medical functions. NAs spent considerable time on both difficult and easy medical tasks in the outpatient department.

Laboratory Personnel

Of those interviewed, 10 percent were employed as laboratory technicians at four of the five hospitals.[5] All twenty-six respondents in this field completed a questionnaire on the functions of general laboratory technicians. In addition to general laboratory work, functions were defined in the specialized areas of

Responses to Patient Care Questionnaire
Sample Questions

Table 17. Percentage of Physicians, Registered Nurses, Nurse Practitioners, and Pediatric Nurse Practitioners Performing Each Function from the Patient Care Questionnaire, and the Percentage of Total Working Time Spent on Each Function by Those Who Perform the Function

Functions	Physician		Registered Nurse		Nurse practitioner		Pediatric nurse practitioner	
	Percentage of group performing each of functions	Percentage of total time spent working on functions	Percentage of group performing each of functions	Percentage of total time spent working on functions	Percentage of group performing each of functions	Percentage of total time spent working on functions	Percentage of group performing each of functions	Percentage of total time spent working on functions
1. Straightening up and cleaning patient's immediate furniture, nurses' stations, utility rooms (GN1)*	55.6	.19	100.0	1.97	100.0	.18	100.0	.35
13. Serving emotional support to patients; entertaining patients (particularly children) (GN 45)*	77.8	1.98	100.0	2.48	100.0	2.78	100.0	3.14
17. Arranging for patient's admission into hospital	66.7	.54	18.2	.12	100.0	.77	33.3	.18
85. Examining heart for abnormal sounds, e.g., murmurs or extra beats	100.0	.51	40.9	.16	100.0	.65	100.0	.58
92. Examining muscles for strength, size, tone, tenderness	100.0	.47	27.3	.13	100.0	.31	100.0	.56
195. Giving intravenous injections	77.8	.28	77.3	.58	50.0	.07	33.3	.24

22_. Treatment regimen for sprains	**55.6**	59.1	.17	50.0	.11	33.3	.09
268. Performing closed chest cardiac massage (GN 46c)*	77.8	59.1	.10	100.0	.18	33.3	.08
Total number of individuals interviewed	9	22	2		3		

Source: *Utilization of Health Personnel: A Five Hospital Study*, Vol. 2, appendix, table A9, pp. A67–A98.

*(GN) indicates those functions taken from the general nursing questionnaire.

Table 18. Patient Care Summary Table
Percentage of Time Spent on Each Group of Functions

Functions by groups	Physicians	Nurse practioners			RNs
		NP	PNP		
Group 1 (1-51)	40.0	23.4	30.6		41.2
Group 2 (52-112)	29.0	42.0	47.3		20.4
Group 3 (113-156)	11.0	9.4	8.9		6.4
Group 4 (157-195)	5.0	3.7	5.2		10.9
Group 5 (196-210)	3.0	.8	1.1		7.1
Group 6 (211-245)	2.0	4.4	.4		7.0
Group 7 (246-255)	6.0	14.9	6.2		4.8
Group 8 (256-279)	4.0	1.5	.3		2.2
Number interviewed:	9	2	3		22

Source: *Utilization of Health Personnel: A Five Hospital Study*, Vol. 2, calculated from table A9, appendix, pp. A67-A98.

bacteriology, chemistry, hematology, histology, urinalysis, blood bank, and cytology.

At each of the four hospitals at which these respondents were employed, most laboratory personnel performed all general functions. At Bacchus Hospital, laboratory personnel were classified as senior, junior, and assistant. Only slight variations in the allotment of time on general laboratory functions could be found between these three employee categories.

The technicians employed in laboratories with limited facilities and only modest workloads tended to perform functions simultaneously in most of the specialties noted above. At the larger institutions, such as Bacchus, the variety and volume of work were much greater. The specialty procedures were assigned on a rotating basis. Over any year, all laboratory workers at the larger hospitals also tended to perform all laboratory tasks, regardless of the degree of complexity.

Many of the laboratory procedures were very repetitive and a number of respondents said they were bored. This was as true of the highly trained performers as of the less highly trained personnel.

X-ray Technicians

Of the 257 interviewed, 16 respondents, or 6 percent of the sample, were employed as x-ray technicians at four of the five hospitals.[6] The greatest bulk of time appeared to be spent on two functions,[7] (1) preparing and positioning patient on x-ray table and (2) taking a routine x-ray. Bacchus Hospital employed 8 of the x-ray technicians in the sample. All 8 performed both of these functions, spending 23.4 percent of their total working time on preparing and positioning patients and 8.6 percent taking routine x-rays.

The functions specific to x-ray technician are few (eighteen separate tasks on our questionnaire), and the degree of technical difficulty appears to be modest. Prolonged formal education or training for this job does not appear to be necessary.

Inhalation Therapists

Twelve of the respondents, or 4.6 percent of the sample, were employed as inhalation therapists at three of the five hospitals. All performers appeared to devote a substantial amount of time to one function — care of Bird and Bennet respirators. At Bacchus Hospital, the six inhalation therapy technicians all performed this function and spent 20.4 percent of their time at it.

Before the 1950s inhalation therapy did not exist as a separate occupation. The functions that these technicians perform were carried out by RNs, aides, or anesthesiologists — or the tasks did not exist. According to the *Occupational Outlook Handbook, 1976-77,* there were thirty-eight thousand people employed as inhalation therapists in the United States in 1974, and openings in this field were expected to increase at a much faster rate than the average for all occupations.[8] This same government publication also reported that inhalation therapists with advanced training and education could expect to do very well in supervisory and teaching positions.

EKG Technicians

Three of the 257 formal interviews were with electrocardiograph technicians at three of the five hospitals.[9] In 1974 there were approximately eleven thousand persons employed as EKG technicians in the United States. The three EKG technicians included in our study were typical of persons working in this field. They were trained on the job by hospital cardiologists and generally performed all functions associated with electrocardiographs.

Psychiatric Nursing

Two psychiatric registered nurses and one psychiatric aide were included in our sample. All three were employed at one of the five hospitals.[10] The RNs and the NA performed most medical functions and spent similar proportions of time on each. For example, "participating in weekly community meeting with all inpatients" was a function performed by both RNs and by the NA, the former on average spending 6.3 percent of their time on this task, and the latter spending 6.1 percent. From the data collected, it is impossible to infer who is the more highly trained performer, the RN or the NA.

Neighborhood Health Workers

Two neighborhood health workers employed at Elektra Hospital were included in our sample.[11] The neighborhood health centers (NHC) in this community were successful in alleviating a large patient burden from the ambulatory facility of the hospital. The success of the NHCs was in large measure the result of the active participation of the neighborhood health workers and their ability to successfully complete medical functions traditionally fulfilled by RNs or MDs.

Ward Secretaries

Twenty-one respondents, or 8.2 percent of the sample, were employed as ward secretaries in four of the five hospitals.[12] To a surprising extent, ward secretary duties overlap those of the NA, LPN, RN, and MD. For example, at Bacchus Hospital, where nine of the twenty-one ward secretaries were employed, 55.6 percent of them spent 5.8 percent of their time on function 1 (charting vital signs, intake and output, and weights). At Desdemona Hospital three of the four ward secretaries spent an average of 14.1 percent of their time on the same function. At Elektra Hospital both ward secretaries spent an average of 13.5 percent of their time on this function. At these institutions marginal medical functions traditionally performed by more formally trained personnel have been assigned to ward secretaries. This observation is significant because it suggests one way to release more highly skilled personnel for tasks that demand their specialized expertise.

7

Analysis of Background Data

Background data on education, training, and personal experience were collected from respondents at all the hospitals. The data from Cressyda will be discussed separately at the end of this section, because this hospital has an innovative in-service training program (discussed in chapter 5), and results from interviews at Cressyda provide some contrast to the findings from the other hospitals. The first part of the discussion is a description of the background data from Adonis, Bacchus, Desdemona, and Elektra hospitals.

Adonis, Bacchus, Desdemona, and Elektra: Background Data

Of those employed in nursing, the majority of the highly skilled nurses (60.7 percent) were between age eighteen and twenty-five, while the majority of the relatively unskilled nurse's aides (65.7 percent) were over the age of forty-one, and 29 percent were over fifty-six (table 19). This inverse relationship between age and skill level is consistent throughout the sample. Most licensed practical nurses (85.7 percent), all nurse practitioners, all x-ray technicians, and 73 percent of the laboratory technicians interviewed were under forty years of age. Conversely, of those in other less highly skilled occupations, 71.4 percent of ward secretaries, 44.2 percent of medical records personnel, and both operating room aides interviewed were over forty-six. The overwhelming majority of the respondents were female; this is not surprising since, with the exception of doctors, the entire health industry is predominantly female. In our sample, males were well represented in the technical occupations: x-ray technician, inhalation therapy technician, and laboratory technician.

When we questioned those in the sample concerning their educational and training background (tables 20 and 21), we found that 17.1 percent of the nurse's aides had only a grammar school education, and 65.7 percent had not received a high school diploma. Personnel in nine other categories had some high school education but had not graduated. These included workers in the LPN category (21.4 percent) and nurse's aide category (48.6 percent), as well as those in the more technical occupations, such as x-ray technicians (6.3 percent), inhalation therapists (8.3 percent), and laboratory technicians (3.8 percent). In the clerical categories, 11.1 percent of the medical records personnel, 33.3 percent of the ward secretaries, and 50 percent of the unit aides had some high school education, but had not graduated. Although the majority of workers in all categories except nurse's aide and unit aide had a high school diploma, those without a diploma functioned as well on their jobs as did those with diplomas. This suggests that the high school diploma is an arbitrary standard having little relevance to the successful performance of many hosptial jobs.

The varied backgrounds of those in the same category were also apparent. Workers in nine of the categories interviewed had some college. The number of LPNs who had between one and four years of high school was equal to the number who had between one and four years of college. In the nurse's aide category, 11.4 percent of those interviewed had some college.

Among RNs the overwhelming majority, 85.1 percent, had graduated from a three-year diploma school; the remainder had graduated from a four-year college program. Of the LPNs included in the sample, half had completed an eighteen-month program, 21.4 percent a fifteen-month program, 21.4 percent a twelve-month program, and 7.1 had not completed any program.

Table 19. Percentage Distribution of Nurse Practitioners, Pediatric Nurse Practitioners, General Nursing Personnel, Ward Secretaries, Operating Room Personnel, Psychiatry Department Personnel, X-Ray Technicians, Inhalation Therapy Technicians, Laboratory Technicians, EKG Technicians, Neighborhood Health Workers, and Medical Records Librarians by Age[1] and Sex[1]

Age	Nurse practitioner	Pediatric nurse practitioner	General nursing RN	General nursing LPN	General nursing NA	Ward unit sec.	Operating room RN	Operating room Tech.	Operating room NA	Psychiatry Department RN	Psychiatry Department Attn.	X-ray tech.	Inhalation tech.	Laboratory tech.	EKG tech.	Neighborhood health worker	Medical records worker	Unit aide
18-25 years	—	—	60.7	64.3	20.0	23.8	—	60.0	—	100.0	100.0	87.5	75.0	26.9	33.3	—	33.3	—
26-40 years	100.0	100.0	26.8	21.4	14.3	4.8	50.0	40.0	—	—	—	12.5	8.3	46.1	33.3	100.0	22.2	50.0
41-55 years	—	—	10.7	7.1	37.1	28.6	25.0	—	—	—	—	—	—	26.9	33.3	—	22.2	50.0
56 and over	—	—	1.8	7.1	28.6	42.8	25.0	—	100.0	—	—	—	16.7	—	—	—	22.2	—
Sex																		
Female	100.0	100.0	100.0	100.0	97.1	100.0	100.0	80.0	50.0	100.0	—	75.0	41.7	92.3	100.0	100.0	88.8	100.0
Male	—	—	—	—	2.8	—	—	20.0	50.0	—	100.0	25.0	58.3	7.7	—	—	11.1	—
Total number of individuals interviewed	2	4	56	14	35	21	4	5	2	2	1	16	12	26	3	2	9	2

Source: Utilization of Health Personnel: A Five Hospital Study, Vol. 2., table A42, p. 199.

[1]May not add to 100 percent because of rounding.

Adonis, Bacchus, Desdemona, Elektra

Table 20. Percentage Distribution of X-Ray Technicians, Inhalation Therapy Technicians, Laboratory Technicians, EKG Technicians, Medical Records Librarians, and Neighborhood Health Workers by Educational and Occupational Training

Educational and occupational training	X-ray tech.	Inhala-tion tech.	Labo-ratory tech.	EKG tech.	Medical records	Neighbor-hood health workers
High school: No high school						
1-4 years	6.3	8.3	3.8	—	11.1	50.0
Diploma received or equivalent	93.7	91.7	96.2	100.0	88.8	50.0
College: 1-4 years (or scattered courses)	81.3	33.3	7.7	33.3	—	—
Diploma received	—	—	30.8	—	33.3	—
Graduate school						
2-year diploma school: Completed						
Not completed						
Nurse's aide training						
Military training course	—	—	3.8			
Foreign training course						
Associate's degree: Completed	18.8	—	11.5			
Not completed	6.3	—	3.8			
College-based, X-ray training program: Completed						
Not completed	—	—	7.7			
Hospital-based training program: Completed	—	—	11.5	33.3		
Not completed	—	—	3.8			
Technical school: Completed						
Not completed						
Formal on-the-job training: At another hospital						
At this hospital						
Informal on-the-job training: At another hospital	31.7	—	3.8	—	11.1	50.0
At this hospital	6.3	66.7	30.8	33.3	44.4	100.0

	NP	PNP	RN	LPN	Nurse's aide	Ward unit secretary	Unit aide
Professional certification: RN	—	8.3	15.4	33.3	—	—	—
R.T., I.R.T., A.R.R.T.	—	8.3	—	—	—	—	—
Still in training	—	16.7	3.8	—	—	—	—
General lab diploma	—	—	11.5	—	—	—	—
ASCP, MT, CLA	—	—	—	100.0	—	—	—
None exists for occupation	—	—	3.8	—	—	—	—
Other	56.3	—	65.4	—	—	—	—
No	43.7	91.7	11.5	—	22.2	—	50.0
Presently enrolled in education institution	—	—	—	—	100.0	—	—
Expects to enroll in an educational institution	—	—	—	—	—	—	—
Specialized training in medical area	12.5	—	—	—	—	—	—
Total number of individuals interviewed	16	12	26	3	9	—	2

Source: *Utilization of Health Personnel: A Five Hospital Study,* Vol. 2., table A43, p. A200.

Adonis, Bacchus, Desdemona, Elektra

Table 21. Percentage Distribution of Nurse Practitioners, Pediatric Nurse Practitioners, Registered Nurses, Licensed Practical Nurses, Nurse's Aides, and Ward Secretaries by Level of Education and Occupational Training

Education and occupational training	NP	PNP	RN	LPN	Nurse's aide	Ward unit secretary	Unit aide
High school: Grammar school, no h.s.	—	—	—	—	17.1	—	—
High school, 1–4 years	—	—	—	21.4	48.6	33.3	50.0
High school, degree received or equivalent	100.0	100.0	100.0	78.6	28.6	66.6	50.0
College: 1–4 years (no 4-year degree)	—	25.0	25.0	21.4	8.6	28.6	—
degree	50.0	75.0	16.1	—	2.9	4.7	—
all with any college	50.0	100.0	41.1	21.4	11.4	33.3	—

(continued on p. 92)

Table 21 (continued)

Graduate school							
Diploma schools: 3-year diploma school completed	50.0	—	85.1	—	—	—	—
3-year diploma school not completed	—	—	1.8	—	—	—	—
LPN 12-month completed	—	—	—	21.4	—	—	—
LPN 15-month completed	—	—	—	21.4	—	4.7	—
LPN 18-month completed	—	—	—	50.0	—	—	—
LPN not completed	—	—	—	7.1	5.7	—	—
Military training course	—	—	—	—	2.9	—	—
Foreign training course	—	—	5.4	—	8.6	—	—
Formal nurse's aide training: At another hospital	—	—	—	—	8.6	—	—
At this hospital	—	—	—	—	11.4	—	—
Informal on-the-job training: At another hospital	—	—	—	—	2.9	—	—
At this hospital	—	—	1.8	7.1	45.7	33.3	—
Typing, secretarial training, MDTA	—	—	—	—	5.7	—	—
Specialized training in medical area	—	—	1.8	—	2.9	18.9	—
Associate's degree	50.0	75.0	1.8	—	—	—	50.0
Certification: RN	100.0	100.0	98.2	—	—	—	—
LPN	—	—	—	92.9	—	—	—
LPN by waiver	—	—	—	—	—	—	100.0
Foreign certification	—	—	—	—	—	—	—
None exists for occupation	—	—	—	—	97.1	90.2	—
Other	—	—	—	—	2.9	9.4	100.0
Presently enrolled in educational institution	—	—	13.9	—	8.6	—	—
Expects to enroll in educational institution	—	—	1.8	—	5.7	9.4	—
Total number of individuals interviewed	2	4	56	14	35	21	2

Source: *Utilization of Health Personnel: A Five Hospital Study,* Vol. 2, table A44, p. A201.

For those occupations for which there is no formal training, such as nurse's aide, on-the-job training becomes much more important because it is the only preparation the employee receives. About 49 percent of nurse's aides reported receiving some informal on-the-job training, while an additional 20 percent received formal nurse's aide training at the hospital that was employing them. One individual, who was trained in the military, was employed as an NA but spent a significant amount of time doing more sophisticated tasks.

Except for RNs and LPNs, a substantial proportion of those interviewed in each category were not certified. Among laboratory personnel more than 65 percent were not certified. Of the inhalation therapists interviewed, only one (8.5 percent) was certified, although several indicated that they intended to take the exam for certification some time in the future. None of the medical records personnel interviewed and less than 57 percent of the x-ray personnel were certified. It should be emphasized that there is no qualitative difference between the functions performed by certified personnel and those performed by noncertified personnel.

On-the-job training (OJT) seems to play an important role in preparing workers in these occupations. Of the nurse's aides, 20 percent had received formal OJT, but over half (51.4 percent) reported that they had received some informal training on the job. In addition, a third of the ward secretaries and EKG technicians, two-thirds of the inhalation therapists, almost a third of the laboratory technicians, and both neighborhood health workers had received informal OJT.

A high turnover rate is generally thought to characterize employment in the health field, but our data for most occupations do not confirm this (tables 22 and 23). More than half of those interviewed in each of nine occupations had been employed for six years or less. These workers were concentrated in occupations requiring a high level of skill and/or professional training. Conversely, more than half of those in occupations which rely on on-the-job training had been employed for ten or more years. Looking at the entire sample, more than half of those interviewed in fourteen of eighteen occupations had been employed in their present position for less than seven years. All nurse practitioners,

Adonis, Bacchus, Desdemona, Elektra

Table 22. Percentage Distribution of Nurse Practitioners, Pediatric Nurse Practitioners, General Nursing Personnel, Ward Secretaries, Operating Room Personnel, Psychiatry Department Personnel, X-Ray Technicians, Inhalation Therapy Technicians, Laboratory Technicians, EKG Technicians, Neighborhood Health Workers, and Medical Records Librarians by Number of Years at Present Occupation[1]

Years employed	Nurse pract.	Pediat. nurse pract.	General nursing RN	LPN	NA	Unit ward sec.	Operating room RN	Tech.	NA	Psychiatry dept. RN	NA Attn.	X-ray tech.	Inhal. tech.	Lab. tech.	EKG tech.	Neigh. health wkr.	Medical records wkr.	Unit records aide
At present occupation																		
Less than 1 year	100.0	—	14.8	7.1	8.6	9.5	—	—	—	—	—	12.5	25.0	3.8	—	—	22.2	—
1-3 years	—	25.0	39.3	35.7	25.7	33.3	—	40.0	—	100.0	100.0	37.5	33.3	23.0	33.3	100.0	33.3	—
4-6 years	—	50.0	21.4	35.7	17.1	42.8	—	40.0	—	—	—	37.5	33.3	30.7	33.3	—	11.1	50.0
7-9 years	—	25.0	7.1	7.1	11.4	14.3	25.0	—	—	—	—	12.5	—	15.4	33.3	—	—	50.0
10-14 years	—	—	3.6	—	8.6	—	—	—	—	—	—	—	—	7.7	—	—	—	—
15 years and over	—	—	12.5	14.3	28.6	—	75.0	20.0	—	—	—	—	—	19.2	—	—	33.3	—
Not applicable: in training	—	—	—	—	—	—	—	—	100.0	—	—	—	—	—	—	—	—	—
At this hospital																		
Less than 1 year	—	25.0	25.0	14.3	14.3	9.5	—	—	—	50.0	—	18.7	58.3	11.5	—	50.0	33.3	50.0
1-3 years	100.0	75.0	51.8	50.0	31.4	38.1	—	80.0	—	50.0	100.0	43.7	25.0	38.4	66.7	50.0	33.3	50.0
4-6 years	—	—	10.7	28.6	17.1	47.6	—	20.0	—	—	—	31.3	8.3	26.9	—	—	33.3	—
7-9 years	—	—	3.6	7.1	8.6	4.8	25.0	—	—	—	—	6.2	—	7.7	—	—	—	—
10-14 years	—	—	3.6	—	5.7	—	25.0	—	—	—	—	—	8.3	7.7	—	—	—	—
15 years and over	—	—	5.3	—	22.8	—	50.0	—	—	—	—	—	—	7.7	33.3	—	—	—
Not applicable: still in training	—	—	—	—	—	—	—	—	100.0	—	—	—	—	—	—	—	—	—
Total number of individuals interviewed	2	4	56	14	35	21	4	5	2	2	1	16	12	26	3	2	9	2

Source: *Utilization of Health Personnel: A Five Hospital Study,* Vol. 2, table A45, p. A202.

[1]May not add to 100 percent because of rounding.

Adonis, Bacchus, Desdemona, Elektra

Table 23. Percentage Distribution of Allied Health Personnel by Employment in Any Other Health Related Occupation [1]

Employment at any other health related occupations	Nurse pract.	Pediat. nurse pract.	General nursing ward RN	LPN	NA	Unit ward sec.	Operating room RN	Tech	NA	Psychiatry RN	Attn	X-ray tech.	Inhal. tech.	Lab tech.	EKG tech.	Neigh. health worker	Medical records	Unit aide
None	50.0	—	57.1	50.0	60.0	66.7	100.0	40.0	100.0	50.0	100.0	62.5	50.0	57.7	66.7	100.0	77.7	50.0
Aide	—	25.0	25.0	14.3	22.9	19.0	—	40.0	—	—	—	6.2	8.3	26.9	—	—	—	—
Volunteer	—	—	8.9	14.3	8.6	4.8	—	20.0	—	—	—	18.7	8.3	3.8	33.3	—	—	—
Nonmedical hospital-based occupation (e.g., sec., clerk)	—	—	5.4	14.3	2.9	9.5	—	—	—	—	—	6.2	8.3	3.8	—	—	11.1	50.0
Employed in physician's office	—	25.0	—	7.1	2.9	—	—	—	—	—	—	—	8.3	7.7	—	—	—	—
RN	100.0	100.0	—	—	2.9	—	—	—	—	—	—	—	—	—	—	—	—	—
Medical corpsman	—	—	—	—	—	—	—	—	—	—	—	—	—	—	—	—	—	—
Research	—	—	—	—	—	—	—	—	—	—	—	—	—	—	—	—	—	—
Mental health worker	—	—	1.8	—	—	—	—	—	—	—	—	—	8.3	—	—	—	—	—
Teaching in medical field	—	—	—	—	—	—	—	—	—	—	—	—	—	—	—	—	—	—
Practical nurse	—	—	—	—	—	—	—	—	—	50.0	—	—	—	—	—	—	—	—
Embalming	—	—	—	—	—	—	—	—	—	—	—	6.2	8.3	—	—	—	—	—
Other	—	—	1.8	—	—	—	—	—	—	—	—	—	—	—	—	—	11.1	—
Total number of individuals interviewed	2	4	56	14	35	21	4	5	2	2	1	16	12	26	3	2	9	2

Source: *Utilization of Health Personnel: A Five Hospital Study*, Vol. 2, table A46, p. 203.

[1] May not add to 100 percent because of personnel having worked in more than one field or because of rounding.

three of four of the RNs, and half of the inhalation therapists, x-ray technicians, and laboratory technicians had worked at their present position for less than three years.

Since the basic findings of the RPO study indicated the importance of on-the-job training, data were collected on the type and duration of the OJT received (table 24). More than a quarter of all those interviewed reported that no OJT was given (26.8 percent of RNs, 28.6 percent of LPNs, and 20 percent of NAs). In the more technical occupations, the figures were even higher: 41.7 percent of inhalation therapists, 40.3 percent of laboratory technicians, and 33.3 percent of the EKG technicians reported no OJT. The responses for x-ray technicians did not follow this trend. Only 18.7 percent reported no OJT, but 81.2 percent reported none was necessary because they had received prior training in a cooperative work/study program or in a hospital program. The length of these programs ranged from less than a day to six weeks. In the nursing department more than a third of RNs and LPNs received an orientation of between two and four weeks. However, among NAs who had received no other training, the period of OJT was about the same as for RNs and LPNs.

A substantial number of workers in the nursing department received orientation to hospital policies, although relatively few workers in other categories were given it.

Respondents were asked what type of orientation they felt they should have received (table 25), and many workers in all categories thought the orientation they had received was suitable. However, though all NAs agreed that a training program was essential, 20 percent had not received any. Every category thought that informal OJT was necessary, although the degree of consensus on this varied (85.6 of RNs, 64.2 percent of LPNs, but only 25.8 percent of the NAs concurred). These results highlight the different needs of each occupation, depending on skill level and amount of formal training. For example, those trained in RN or LPN programs require more informal orientation to the hospital setting than NAs who receive all their training in formal OJT at the hospital.

All pediatric nurse practitioners (PNPs), operating room RNs and NAs, psychiatric RNs and attendants, neighborhood health workers, and unit aides agreed that OJT was important. Nearly 27

Adonis, Bacchus, Desdemona, Elektra

Table 24. Percentage Distribution of Allied Health Personnel by What They Feel Their Orientation Was[1]

Orientation	Nurse pract.	Pediat. nurse pract.	Ward: General nursing unit — RN	LPN	NA	sec.	Ward: Operating room — RN	Tech.	NA	Ward: Psychiatry — RN	Attn.	X-ray tech.	Inhal. tech.	Lab tech.	EKG tech.	Neigh. health nurse	Medical worker	Medical records	Unit aide
Length of orientation																			
Less than a day	50.0	25.0	1.9	—	2.8	4.8	—	—	—	—	—	—	—	—	15.4	33.3	—	33.3	—
1-5 days	50.0	—	25.0	21.4	14.3	33.3	—	20.0	—	—	—	—	16.7	7.7	—	—	—	22.2	50.0
2-4 weeks	—	25.0	35.7	35.7	40.0	28.6	25.0	—	50.0	50.0	—	—	16.7	11.5	—	—	—	—	50.0
4-6 weeks	—	—	3.6	14.3	14.3	—	25.0	—	50.0	50.0	—	—	—	—	—	—	—	—	—
More than 6 weeks	—	—	3.6	—	8.6	14.3	—	20.0	—	—	—	81.2	8.3	7.7	33.3	—	—	11.1	—
None necessary	—	—	3.6	—	2.8	9.5	25.0	—	—	—	—	—	—	—	—	—	—	—	—
None given	—	—	26.8	28.6	20.0	—	50.0	—	60.0	—	—	18.7	41.7	40.3	33.3	—	—	11.1	—
Type of orientation																			
Introduction to hospital policies	—	—	51.8	42.8	54.3	47.6	20.0	—	—	—	—	—	25.0	23.1	33.3	—	—	—	—
Formal classes in the hospital	—	—	48.2	42.8	54.3	23.8	—	—	50.0	50.0	—	—	25.0	11.5	—	—	—	11.1	50.0
Informal on-the-job training by supervisor	50.0	—	7.1	21.4	54.3	14.3	—	—	50.0	—	—	—	16.7	11.5	—	100.0	—	22.2	—
Informal on-the-job training by fellow worker	—	—	1.8	—	—	33.3	—	—	—	100.0	—	—	16.7	19.2	—	—	—	22.2	—
Informal training (unspecified)	50.0	50.0	35.7	11.4	42.8	—	50.0	20.0	50.0	100.0	—	—	—	3.8	—	—	—	—	100.0

(continued on p. 98)

Table 24 (continued)

Additional training beyond orientation	—	—	—	—	9.5	—	—	—	—	—	—	—	—	—	—	—	—	—
More extensive training to learn more	—	—	—	—	—	—	—	—	—	—	—	—	—	—	—	—	—	—
Continuing in-service program	100.0	—	7.1	—	5.7	9.5	25.0	—	50.0	—	—	16.7	3.8	—	9.5	—	16.7	3.8	—	22.2
Total number of individuals interviewed	2	4	56	14	35	21	4	5	2	2	1	16	12	26	3	2	9	2

Source: *Utilization of Health Personnel: A Five Hospital Study,* Vol. 2, table A47, p. A204.

[1] May not add to 100 percent because of rounding.

Adonis, Bacchus, Desdemona, Elektra

Table 25. Percentage Distribution of Allied Health Personnel by What They Feel Their Orientation Should Be[1]

Orientation / Length of orientation	Nurse pract.	Pediat. nurse pract.	General nursing unit RN	LPN	NA	sec.	Operating room RN	Tech.	NA	Psychiatry RN	NA	Attn.	X-ray tech.	Inhal. tech.	Lab tech.	EKG tech.	Neigh. health worker	Medical Records	Unit aide
Less than a day	25.0	—	—	—	—	—	—	20.0	—	—	—	—	—	—	—	—	—	—	—
1–5 days	—	—	16.1	21.4	8.6	14.3	—	—	—	—	—	—	6.2	16.7	—	—	50.0	11.1	50.0
2–4 weeks	—	—	42.8	35.7	42.8	38.1	—	—	50.0	100.0	—	—	—	8.3	3.8	66.7	50.0	22.2	50.0
4–6 weeks	—	—	7.1	7.1	11.4	9.5	75.0	—	—	—	—	—	—	—	7.7	—	—	—	—
More than 6 weeks	25.0	—	3.6	—	8.6	4.8	25.0	—	20.0	—	—	—	6.2	—	3.8	—	—	22.2	—

None necessary	—	—	1.8	7.1	5.7	—	—	20.0	—	—	—	62.5	8.3	49.0	—	—	—
None given	100.0	50.0	28.6	28.6	—	14.3	—	20.0	50.0	—	100.0	25.0	66.7	35.7	33.3	—	22.2
Type of orientation																	
Introduction to hospital policies	—	—	30.3	14.3	54.3	—	—	40.0	—	—	—	—	8.3	19.3	—	—	—
Formal classes in the hospital	—	—	64.3	21.4	20.0	47.6	25.0	20.0	50.0	50.0	—	—	58.3	19.3	33.3	—	11.1
Informal on-the-job training by supervisor[2]	—	50.0	19.6	42.8	—	23.8	—	—	50.0	—	—	6.2	8.3	42.3	33.3	100.0	33.3
Informal on-the-job training by fellow worker	—	—	25.0	17.8	7.1	20.0	23.8	50.0	20.0	—	100.0	6.2	33.3	19.3	—	—	55.5
Informal on-the-job training (unspecified)	—	25.0	48.2	14.3	5.8	33.3	50.0	20.0	50.0	—	100.0	18.7	25.0	7.7	33.3	—	11.1
Additional training beyond orientation																	
More extensive training to learn more	—	—	1.8	—	17.1	9.5	—	—	—	—	—	—	—	-	—	—	—
Continuing in-service program	100.0	—	26.8	7.1	11.4	19.0	—	—	—	—	—	6.2	8.3	7.7	—	—	11.1
Total number of individuals interviewed	2	4	56	14	35	21	4	5	2	2	1	16	12	26	3	2	9

Source: *Utilization of Health Personnel: A Five Hospital Study,* Vol. 2, table A48, p. 205.

[1] May not add to 100 percent because of rounding.

[2] For nurse's aides, orientation and training are synonymous.

Adonis, Bacchus, Desdemona, Elektra

Table 26. Percentage Distribution of Nurse Practitioners, Pediatric Nurse Practitioners, General Nursing Personnel, Ward Secretaries, Operating Room Personnel, Psychiatry Department Personnel, X-Ray Technicians, Inhalation Therapy Technicians, Laboratory Technicians, EKG Technicians, Neighborhood Health Workers, and Medical Records Librarians by the Formal Level of Education They Feel Should Be Required for Their Field[1]

| Formal Level of education | Nurse pract. | Pediat. nurse pract. | General nursing unit | | | Ward sec. | Operating room | | | Psychiatry | | X-ray tech. | Inhal. tech. | Lab tech. | EKG tech. | Neigh. health tech. | Medical records worker | Unit aide |
			RN	LPN	NA		RN	Tech.	NA	RN	Attn.							
1. No requirement	—	—	—	—	53.9	14.3	50.0	20.0	50.0	—	100.0	—	16.7	—	—	100.0	22.2	100.0
2. High school, no diploma	—	—	—	—	23.0	23.8	—	20.0	50.0	—	—	6.2	8.3	3.8	—	—	—	—
3. High school, diploma	—	—	—	7.1	11.4	38.1	—	40.0	—	—	—	—	—	—	66.7	—	—	—
4. College — varied courses	—	—	—	—	—	—	—	—	—	100.0	—	25.0	25.0	—	—	—	55.5	—
5. College — 2 year-degree	—	—	5.4	—	—	—	—	—	—	—	—	6.2	—	23.1	—	—	—	—
6. College — 4 year-degree	—	—	19.6	—	—	—	—	—	—	—	—	24.6	8.3	26.9	—	—	—	—
7. 3-year diploma school	50.0	25.0	44.6	—	—	—	—	—	—	—	—	—	—	7.7	—	—	—	—
8. 12-month LPN school	—	—	—	28.6	—	25.0	—	—	—	—	—	—	—	—	—	—	—	—
9. 18-month LPN school	—	—	—	42.9	—	—	—	—	—	—	—	—	—	3.8	—	—	—	—
10. College-based training	—	—	—	—	—	—	—	—	—	—	—	6.3	8.3	7.7	—	—	22.2	—

11. Hospital-based training	—	—	—	—	5.7	—	—	20.0	—	—	—	25.0	16.7	7.7	—	—	—	—
12. Depends on individual	50.0	75.0	14.3	21.4	8.6	23.8	25.0	—	—	50.0	—	—	16.7	19.2	33.3	50.0	—	—
13. 3 yr. or B.S. no preference	—	—	16.1	—	—	—	—	—	—	—	—	—	—	—	—	—	—	—
Total number of individuals interviewed	2	4	56	14	35	21	4	5	2	2	1	16	12	26	3	2	9	2

Source: *Utilization of Health Personnel: A Five Hospital Study*, Vol. 2, table A49, P. A206.

[1]May not add to 100 percent because more than one answer was given in some cases.

Adonis, Bacchus, Desdemona, Elektra

Table 27. Percentage Distribution of Allied Health Personnel by Personal Qualities That They Feel Are Important in Their Field or Department

Personal qualities that are felt to be important	Nurse pract.	Pediat. nurse pract.	General nursing			Ward unit sec.	Operating room			Psychiatry		X-ray tech.	Inhal. tech.	Lab tech.	EKG tech.	Neigh. health wkr.	Medical records wkr.	Unit aide
			RN	LPN	NA		RN	Tech.	NA	RN	Attn.							
A liking for people	100.0	25.0	33.9	35.7	45.7	28.6	50.0	—	50.0	100.0	—	56.2	58.3	23.1	33.3	50.0	—	—
Patience	—	50.0	21.4	28.6	25.7	38.1	75.0	40.0	—	—	—	18.7	33.3	15.4	33.3	100.0	55.5	—
Even-temper	—	25.0	17.8	—	2.8	23.8	25.0	60.0	—	—	—	6.2	8.3	3.8	66.7	—	11.1	—
Maturity	—	25.0	26.8	35.7	14.3	14.3	25.0	—	—	50.0	100.0	25.0	8.3	34.6	33.3	50.0	44.4	—
Compassion	—	—	28.6	35.7	11.4	4.8	—	—	—	50.0	—	25.0	25.0	11.5	—	—	—	—
Politeness	—	—	1.8	—	11.4	33.3	25.0	—	—	—	—	—	—	—	33.3	—	—	—
Friendliness	50.0	—	16.1	14.3	14.3	33.3	25.0	—	—	—	—	6.2	8.3	15.4	—	—	11.1	—
Conscientiousness	—	—	14.3	—	—	9.5	—	40.0	—	—	—	6.2	16.7	15.4	33.3	—	33.3	—
Intelligence	—	25.0	14.3	—	2.8	9.5	—	—	—	—	—	18.7	25.0	—	—	50.0	—	—
Common sense	—	25.0	16.1	—	2.8	9.5	25.0	—	—	—	—	—	—	7.7	33.3	—	—	—
Flexibility	—	—	10.7	7.1	2.8	4.8	25.0	—	50.0	—	—	12.5	—	—	—	—	11.1	—
Efficiency	—	—	7.1	—	—	—	25.0	—	—	—	—	—	—	—	—	—	—	—
Professional attitude	50.0	25.0	21.4	14.3	20.0	9.5	50.0	20.0	50.0	100.0	—	18.7	50.0	50.0	66.7	—	33.3	—
Dexterity	50.0	50.0	7.1	—	8.5	14.3	—	40.0	—	—	—	15.4	—	15.4	—	—	33.3	50.0
Accuracy	—	—	—	—	—	—	—	—	—	—	—	6.2	16.7	19.2	—	—	—	—
Eagerness	—	25.0	8.9	7.1	—	—	—	20.0	—	50.0	—	6.2	16.7	11.5	—	—	—	—
Stamina	—	—	7.1	7.1	—	—	—	20.0	—	—	—	6.2	8.3	7.7	—	—	11.1	—
Leadership	—	—	5.3	7.1	—	—	—	20.0	—	—	—	6.2	8.3	—	—	—	—	—
None in particular	—	—	—	7.1	—	—	—	—	50.0	—	—	—	—	—	—	—	—	50.0
Total number of individuals interviewed	2	4	56	14	35	21	4	5	2	2	1	16	12	26	3	2	9	2

Source: *Utilization of Health Personnel: A Five Hospital Study*, Vol. 2, table A50, P. A207.

percent of the RNs, over 11 percent of the NAs, and 19 percent of ward secretaries suggested that a continuing in-service program would be of value. In addition, 17.1 percent of the NAs and 9.5 percent of the ward secretaries felt that their initial training should have been more extensive.

Workers were also asked to assess the amount of formal education that should be required for their jobs (table 26). Most significant were the responses from workers in occupations for which formal certification is not required. Over 50 percent of the NAs, more than 14 percent of the ward secretaries, 20 percent of the operating room technicians, and both neighborhood health workers thought that there should be no education requirement. Others in these categories thought that some high school education would be useful. Approximately 40 percent of ward secretaries and operating room technicians thought that a high school diploma was necessary. Many stated that this depended on the individual; they felt that the way they were trained was good for them, though not necessarily the only way to be trained.

Table 27 reports the personal qualities that were felt to be important in the worker's field. Those interviewed most often stated that patience, maturity, and a liking for people were necessary qualities to function well in these jobs. This offers no new information, but it does reflect the attitude held by most workers in the health field.

When questioned about the relevance of their previous experience and training to their present jobs, workers in all categories stressed practical experience (table 28). Respondents in nine categories said practical experience prepared them more than anything else. For example, NAs thought that practical experience had provided them with nearly half of the skills needed to perform their job. Even RNs, for whom formal training plays a more important role, indicated that practical experience was about equal in importance to professional training.

The original pilot study done by the Center for Medical Manpower Studies has shown the importance of upward mobility. Job satisfaction can be as much a function of the potential for advancement as it is of wages and working conditions. When workers were asked to assess the possibilities for promotion within

Adonis, Bacchus, Desdemona, Elektra

Table 28. Ranking Distribution of Allied Health Personnel by Extent to Which the Following Experiences Prepared Them for the Function They Are Presently Performing

Extent to which the following prepared them for their functions	Nurse pract.	Pediatric nurse pract.	General nursing ward RN	LPN	NA	Unit sec.	Operating room RN	Tech.	NA	Psychiatry RN	Attn.	X-ray tech.	Inhal. tech.	Lab tech.	EKG tech.	Neigh. health worker	Medical records	Unit aide
High school	—	1.3	12.3	10.0	12.0	27.4	2.5	6.5	35.0	4.5	—	13.0	5.8	12.0	20.0	—	18.5	—
College	10.0	11.3	9.0	2.1	2.4	2.4	—	—	—	33.6	—	22.9	5.8	13.9	5.0	—	3.9	—
Vocational/ technical training	—	—	1.0	2.1	1.1	5.2	—	—	—	—	—	.3	—	5.4	—	—	—	—
On-the-job training	—	7.5	6.2	6.8	33.3	19.7	—	10.0	—	13.7	—	38.9	53.3	20.2	30.0	20.0	47.8	—
Professional training	22.5	43.8	36.4	51.8	4.1	2.2	53.7	54.3	—	—	50.0	3.1	3.3	14.7	10.0	—	1.7	—
Practical experiences	67.5	30.0	34.7	27.1	45.9	43.1	43.7	29.2	65.0	48.2	50.0	21.7	31.7	33.8	35.0	62.5	22.6	100.0
Other	—	6.2	—	—	1.4	—	—	—	—	—	—	—	—	—	—	17.5	5.6	—
Total number of individuals interviewed	2	4	56	14	35	21	4	5	2	2	1	16	12	26	3	2	9	2

Source: *Utilization of Health Personnel: A Five Hospital Study,* Vol. 2, table A52, p. A210.

their occupations without further education or training (table 29), their responses supported our findings in *Hiring Standards for Paramedical Manpower* and in *Restructuring Paramedical Occupations:*

Obviously not everyone has a burning desire to climb some real or mythical occupational ladder. Many persons interviewed had become conditioned to their occupational status and realized the present realistic limits to any upward mobility.[1]

Workers in eleven occupations thought that it was possible to advance, but it was mostly workers in higher-skilled jobs who felt this way. Seventy-five percent of PNPs, 53.6 percent of RNs, 56.2 percent of x-ray technicians, and 66.6 percent of EKG technicians thought there was some vertical mobility, though not all wanted to advance. In contrast, all LPNs thought that their job was dead-end, as did 94.1 percent of NAs, 76.2 percent of ward secretaries, 75 percent of operating room RNs, all operating room technicians, psychiatric attendants, and neighborhood health workers. Even among RNs, who have a high level of skill, 37.5 percent viewed their job as dead-end. Few thought there was potential for upward mobility if they left the hospital. Restricted upward mobility is endemic to the entire health industry and is further complicated by licensing laws and limited lateral mobility.

Many of those interviewed planned to remain with the present employer (table 30). This was especially true of those in less-skilled occupations (60 percent of NAs, 76.2 percent of ward secretaries, 100 percent of NAs in the operating room, 100 percent of neighborhood health workers, and 77.7 percent of medical records personnel). Others expected to leave although they had not yet made specific plans to do so. Some workers interviewed had definite plans to leave; within general nursing, this category included 28.6 percent of RNs, 21.4 percent of LPNs, and 25.7 percent of NAs. Those who planned to remain most often cited satisfaction with the work and liking their co-workers as their reasons for wanting to stay.

Adonis, Bacchus, Desdemona, Elektra

Table 29. Percentage Distribution of Allied Health Personnel by the Occupational Level They Can Realistically Hope to Attain with Their Present Educational and Professional Training[1]

Occupational Level they can realistically hope to attain	Nurse practitioner	Pediatric nurse practitioner	General Nursing RN	General Nursing LPN	General Nursing NA	Ward sec.	Operating room RN	Operating room LPN	Operating room NA	Psychiatry RN	Psychiatry Attn.	X-ray	Inhal. tech.	Lab tech.	EKG tech.	Neigh. health worker	Medical records	Unit aide
Can go higher and would like to	—	—	25.0	—	—	4.8	—	—	—	—	—	12.5	8.3	3.8	—	—	22.2	—
Can go higher, but would not like to	—	25.0	3.6	—	—	—	—	—	—	100.0	—	18.7	—	—	—	—	—	—
Can go higher, but unclear if respondent would like to or not	—	50.0	—	—	2.8	14.3	25.0	—	—	—	—	25.0	16.6	23.1	66.6	—	22.2	50.0
Total: can go higher	—	75.0	53.6	—	2.8	19.0	25.0	—	—	100.0	—	56.2	25.0	26.9	66.6	—	44.4	50.0
Dead end, but would like to go higher	—	25.0	12.5	50.0	22.8	14.3	25.0	—	—	—	—	—	—	7.7	—	—	22.2	—
Dead end, but satisfied	—	—	—	7.1	22.8	28.6	50.0	20.0	—	—	—	—	—	3.8	—	—	—	—
Dead end, but unclear if respondent is satisfied or not	66.7	—	25.0	42.8	48.5	33.3	—	80.0	50.0	—	100.0	25.0	4.7	38.5	—	100.0	22.2	—
Total: dead end	66.7	25.0	37.5	100.0	94.1	76.2	75.0	100.0	50.0	—	100.0	25.0	4.7	50.0	—	100.0	44.4	—
Would have to leave hospital to go higher and might consider it	—	—	—	—	2.8	—	—	—	—	—	—	6.2	3.8	—	—	—	11.1	—
Would have to leave hospital to go higher, but does not intend to	33.3	—	—	—	—	—	—	—	—	—	—	12.5	3.8	—	—	—	—	—
Total: must leave to advance	33.3	—	—	—	2.8	—	—	—	—	—	—	18.7	7.7	—	—	—	11.1	—
Generally unsure	—	—	8.9	—	—	4.8	—	—	50.0	—	—	—	8.3	—	33.3	—	—	—
No response	—	—	—	—	—	—	—	—	—	—	—	—	8.3	—	—	—	—	—
Total number of individuals interviewed	3	4	56	14	35	21	4	5	2	2	1	16	12	26	3	2	9	2

Source: *Utilization of Health Personnel: A Five Hospital Study,* Vol. 2, table A51, pp. 208-9.

[1] May not add to 100 percent because of rounding or because more than one answer was given.

Cressyda: Background Data

Interviews at Cressyda included RNs, LPNs, and four categories of NAs (nursing technician, senior nursing technician, nursing assistant, and senior nursing assistant). Table 31 shows the age and sex distribution of those interviewed. Eighty percent of RNs and 66.7 percent of LPNs were less than twenty-five years of age. In the NA categories, there was a wider age distribution: nursing assistants and senior nursing assistants were younger as a group than those in the more advanced technician categories. All respondents were female with the exception of two nursing technicians.

With respect to educational level (table 32), a sizable number in each category had less than a high school diploma. This is especially true of those interviewed in the NA categories where half of the workers had not completed high school. The turnover rate for nurse's aides at Cressyda (table 33) appears to be less than that in the other four hospitals. Over 60 percent of the nursing technicians and two-thirds of the senior nursing assistants had worked between four and nine years at the hospital. This is an indication that the occupational ladder provided by the hospital may contribute to a more stable work force.

Table 34 reflects the extensiveness of the in-service training. In addition, 40 percent of RNs and 33.3 percent of LPNs received OJT. When asked what type of orientation they thought was appropriate (table 35), nearly all who were interviewed stressed the importance of OJT, including all NAs, 80 percent of RNs, and 66.7 percent of LPNs.

Opinions on the importance of a high school diploma were mixed (table 36). Among those interviewed in the two lower categories of NAs, 66.7 percent of senior nursing assistants and 50 percent of the nursing assistants did not feel a high school diploma was necessary to perform their job. However, 80 percent of the senior nursing technicians thought that a high school diploma was important. Respondents in all categories felt they were prepared for their present function in large measure by practical experience, and all valued on-the-job training (table 37).

Adonis, Bacchus, Desdemona, Elektra

Table 30. Percentage Distribution of Allied Health Personnel by Their Plans for Future Employment and Their Reasons[1]

Future plans and reasons for them	Nurse pract.	Pediatric nurse pract.	General nursing			Ward unit sec.	Operating room			Psychiatry			X-ray tech.	Inhal. tech.	Lab tech.	EKG tech.	Neigh. health worker	Medical records	Unit aide
			RN	LPN	NA		RN	Tech.	NA	RN	RN	Attn.							
Plan to remain at this hospital	50.0	75.0	46.4	28.6	60.0	76.2	100.0	40.0	100.0	—	—	—	31.2	58.3	50.0	66.7	100.0	77.7	50.0
Plan to leave	50.0	25.0	28.6	21.4	25.7	9.5	—	40.0	—	—	—	—	37.5	25.0	15.4	—	—	11.1	—
Plan to stay indefinitely	—	—	10.7	35.7	5.7	4.8	—	20.0	—	100.0	—	—	12.5	—	15.4	33.3	—	11.1	50.0
No plans/unsure	—	—	12.5	14.3	5.7	9.5	—	—	—	—	100.0	—	18.7	8.3	15.4	—	—	—	—
No response	—	—	1.8	—	—	—	—	—	—	—	—	—	—	8.3	3.8	—	—	—	—
Reason for remaining																			
1. Like the work/people	50.0	50.0	28.6	14.3	71.4	42.8	25.0	—	—	—	—	—	12.5	8.3	23.1	33.3	100.0	66.6	—
2. Convenience	—	—	—	—	—	9.5	75.0	20.0	—	—	—	—	—	—	—	—	—	11.1	—
3. Settled here	—	—	7.1	5.7	—	4.8	—	—	—	—	—	—	—	—	—	—	—	—	—
4. Employee/retirement benefits	—	—	—	—	—	—	—	—	50.0	—	—	—	—	—	—	—	—	—	—
5. Good salary	—	—	5.3	—	2.8	—	—	—	—	—	—	—	6.2	—	3.8	—	—	—	—
6. No place else to go	—	—	3.5	—	2.8	—	—	—	—	—	—	—	—	—	3.8	—	—	11.1	—
7. Other/none	50.0	25.0	1.8	14.3	8.6	19.0	—	40.0	50.0	100.0	100.0	—	25.0	50.0	15.4	66.7	—	11.1	100.0

Reasons for leaving																		
1. Personal reasons	—	25.0	5.3	7.1	2.8	4.8	—	20.0	—	—	—	—	—	3.8	—	11.1	—	—
2. Temporary employment	—	—	3.5	—	—	—	—	—	—	—	—	—	8.3	—	—	—	—	—
3. Dissatisfied with working conditions	—	—	8.9	—	8.6	—	—	—	—	—	—	6.2	—	3.8	—	—	—	—
4. Cannot advance here	—	—	3.5	—	2.8	—	—	—	—	—	—	—	—	—	—	—	—	—
5. Returning to school	—	—	1.8	7.1	2.8	—	—	—	—	—	—	—	—	—	—	—	—	—
6. Completion of alternative service	—	—	1.8	—	—	—	—	—	—	—	—	—	—	—	—	—	—	—
7. Other/none	50.0	—	10.7	7.1	8.6	9.5	—	20.0	—	—	—	31.2	16.6	3.8	—	—	—	—
Total number of individuals interviewed	2	4	56	14	35	21	4	5	2	2	1	16	12	26	3	2	9	2

Source: *Utilization of Health Personnel: A Five Hospital Study*, Vol. 2, table A53, p. A211.

[1]May not add to 100 percent because of rounding or because more than one answer was given.

Cressyda

Table 31. Percentage Distribution of General Nursing Personnel, Senior Nursing Technicians, Nursing Technicians, Senior Nursing Assistants, and Nursing Assistants by Age[1] and Sex[1]

| Age | General nursing | | Senior nursing technician | Nursing technician | Senior nursing assistant | Nursing assistant |
	RN	LPN				
18-25 years	80.0	66.7	—	25.0	33.3	100.0
26-40 years	—	—	60.0	37.5	66.7	—
41-55 years	20.0	33.3	40.0	25.0	—	—
56 and over	—	—	—	12.5	—	—
Sex						
Female	100.0	100.0	80.0	87.5	100.0	100.0
Male	—	—	20.0	12.5	—	—
Total number of individuals interviewed	5	3	5	8	3	8

Source: *Utilization of Health Personnel: A Five Hospital Study*, Vol. 2, table A79, p. A237.

[1]May not add up to 100 percent because of rounding.

Cressyda

Table 32. Percentage Distribution of Registered Nurses, Licensed Practical Nurses, Senior Nursing Technicians, Nursing Technicians, Senior Nursing Assistants, Nursing Assistants, by Level of Education and Occupational Training

	RN	LPN	Senior nursing tech	Nursing tech	Senior nursing ass't	Nursing ass't
Education and occupational training						

High School: Grammar school, no h.s.	—	—	—	—	—	—
High school, 1-4 years	20.0	33.3	60.0	50.0	33.3	50.0
High school, degree received or equivalent	80.0	33.3	20.0	50.0	66.7	50.0
College: 1-4 years	—	33.3	—	12.5	—	—
Degree	20.0	—	—	—	—	—
All with any college	—	—	—	12.5	—	—
Graduate School	100.0	—	—	—	—	—
Diploma schools: 3-year diploma school completed	—	66.7	—	—	—	—
3-year diploma school not completed	—	—	—	—	—	—
LPN 12-month completed	—	—	—	—	—	—
LPN 15-month completed	—	—	—	—	—	—
LPN 18-month completed	—	—	—	—	—	—
LPN not completed	—	—	—	—	—	12.5
Military training course	—	33.3	—	—	—	—
Foreign training course	—	33.3	—	—	—	—
Formal nurse's aid training: At another hospital	20.0	33.3	20.0	37.5	33.3	—
At this hospital	60.0	—	60.0	87.5	33.3	100.0
Informal on-the-job training: At another hospital	—	—	—	—	66.7	—
At this hospital	—	—	—	—	—	12.5
Typing, secretarial training, MDTA	—	—	—	—	—	—
Specialized training in medical area	20.0	—	—	12.5	—	—
Associate's degree	100.0	—	—	—	—	—
Certification: RN	—	100.0	—	—	—	—
LPN	—	—	—	—	—	—
LPN by waiver	—	—	—	—	—	—
Foreign certification	—	—	—	—	—	—
None exists for occupation	—	—	—	—	—	—
Other	20.0	—	20.0	—	—	—
Presently enrolled in educational institution	—	—	—	12.5	—	12.5
Expects to enroll in educational institution	—	—	—	—	—	—
Total number of individuals interviewed	5	3	5	8	3	8

Source: *Utilization of Health Personnel: A Five Hospital Study*, Vol. 2, table A80, p. A238.

Cressyda

Table 33. Percentage Distribution of Registered Nurses, Licensed Practical Nurses, Senior Nursing Technicians, Nursing Technicians, Senior Nursing Assistants, Nursing Assistants by Number of Years at Present Occupation[1]

Years employed at present occupation	RN	LPN	Senior nursing technician	Nursing technician	Senior Nursing assistant	Nursing assistant
Less than 1 year	20.0	—	—	—	—	75.0
1-3 years	40.0	66.7	20.0	25.0	33.3	12.5
4-6 years	20.0	—	20.0	50.0	33.3	12.5
7-9 years	—	—	20.0	12.5	33.3	—
10-14 years	—	—	40.0	—	—	—
15 years and over	20.0	33.3	—	12.5	—	—
Not applicable: in training	—	—	—	—	—	—
Years employed at this hospital						
Less than 1 year	20.0	—	20.0	12.5	33.3	75.0
1-3 years	40.0	66.7	—	25.0	33.3	25.0
4-6 years	20.0	—	40.0	37.5	33.3	—
7-9 years	—	—	20.0	25.0	—	—
10-14 years	—	—	20.0	—	—	—
15 years and over	20.0	33.3	—	—	—	—
Not applicable: still in training	—	—	—	—	—	—
Total number of individuals interviewed	5	3	5	8	3	8

Source: *Utilization of Health Personnel: A Five Hospital Study*, Vol. 2, table A81, p.A239.

[1]May not add to 100 percent because of rounding.

The results on table 38 show that, unlike workers at other hospitals, those at Cressyda felt there were opportunities to advance. All RNs, nursing assistants, and senior nursing assistants, as well at 75 percent of nursing technicians, thought they could advance. On the other hand, most LPNs (66.6 percent) and senior nursing technicians (60 percent) felt that their jobs were dead-end. None of the personnel in the latter two categories was clearly dissatisfied with this situation; it is relevant to note that all senior nursing technicians said they intended to stay at the hospital and only one-third of the LPNs had definite plans to leave (table 39).

Comparison of Background Data

In comparing the background data from Cressyda with that from other hospitals, several contrasts emerge. With respect to age, the inverse relationship between age and skill level seen in the nursing categories at the four hospitals does not appear among nurse's aides at Cressyda. Instead, there is a direct relationship between age and skill level. Although most RNs and LPNs at Cressyda are under twenty-five years of age, a relatively large percentage in both categories are over forty. At the other hospitals only a small fraction of the sample of RNs and LPNs were older than forty.

Another difference appears in the turnover rates. There is a tendency for nursing personnel at Cressyda to have worked longer at their present occupations than workers at the other hospitals. However, it should be kept in mind that Cressyda is the major employer in a large rural area and the stability of its work force is undoubtedly due in part to the scarcity of alternate employers, especially in the health field. Probably the most striking difference between Cressyda and the other hospitals is in the respondents' views of the possibilities for advancement. Personnel at Cressyda generally thought they could advance if they wished, while at the other hospitals most respondents thought they were in dead-end jobs and many were clearly dissatisfied about it.

Cressyda

Table 34. Percentage Distribution of Allied Health Personnel by Type of Orientation They Received[1]

Orientation	RN	LPN	Senior nursing technician	Nursing technician	Senior nursing assistant	Nursing assistant
Length of orientation						
Less than a day	—	—	—	12.5	—	—
1-5 days	20.0	—	20.0	12.5	33.3	—
2-4 weeks	20.0	33.3	—	12.5	—	—
4-6 weeks	—	—	20.0	25.0	—	—
More than 6 weeks	—	—	40.0	25.0	—	100.0
None necessary	40.0	—	20.0	12.5	66.7	—
None given	20.0	66.7	—	—	—	—
Type of orientation						
Introduction to hospital policies	40.0	33.3	80.0	87.5	100.0	100.0
Formal classes in the hospital	—	—	40.0	62.5	100.0	100.0
Informal on-the-job training by supervisor[2]	40.0	33.3	60.0	62.5	100.0	100.0
Informal on-the-job training by fellow worker	—	—	—	—	—	—
On-the-job training (unspecified)	—	—	—	—	—	—
Additional training beyond orientation						
More extensive training to learn more	—	—	—	—	—	—
Continuing in-service program	100.0	100.0	100.0	100.0	100.0	100.0
Total no. of individuals interviewed	5	3	5	8	3	8

Source: *Utilization of Health Personnel: A Five Hospital Study*, Vol. 2, table A83, p. A241.

[1] May not add to 100 percent because of rounding.

[2] For Nurse's aides, orientation and training are synonymous.

Cressyda

Table 35. Percentage Distribution of Allied Health Personnel by What They Feel Their Orientation Should be[1]

Orientation	RN	LPN	Senior nursing technician	Nursing technician	Senior nursing assistant	Nursing assistant
Length of orientation						
Less than a day	—	—	—	—	—	—
1-5 days	20.0	33.3	40.0	—	—	—
2-4 weeks	—	—	—	—	—	—
4-6 weeks	—	—	—	25.0	—	25.0
More than 6 weeks	—	—	—	—	—	—
None necessary	—	—	—	—	—	—
None given	80.0	66.7	60.0	75.0	100.0	75.0
Type of orientation						
Introduction to hospital policies	20.0	33.3	—	—	—	—
Formal classes in the hospital	100.0	33.3	60.0	87.5	100.0	100.0
Informal on-the-job training by supervisor[2]	20.0	33.3	—	—	—	—
Informal on-the-job training by fellow worker	—	—	—	—	—	—
On-the-job training (unspecified)	80.0	66.7	100.0	100.0	100.0	100.0
Additional training beyond orientation						
More extensive training to learn more	—	—	—	—	—	—
Continuing in-service program	—	33.3	—	—	—	37.5
Total no. of individuals interviewed	5	3	5	8	3	8

Source: *Utilization of Health Personnel: A Five Hospital Study,* Vol. 2, table A84, p. A242.

[1]May not add to 100 percent because of rounding.
[2]For Nurse's aides, orientation and training are synonymous.

Cressyda

Table 36. Percentage Distribution of Registered Nurses, Licensed Practical Nurses, Senior Nursing Technicians, Nursing Technicians, Senior Nursing Assistants, Nursing Assistants by the Formal Level of Education They Feel Should Be Required in Their Field[1]

Formal level of education	RN	LPN	Senior nursing technician	Nursing technician	Senior nursing assistant	Nursing assistant
1. No requirement	—	—	20.0	12.5	—	—
2. High school, no diploma	—	—	—	—	—	—
3. High school, diploma	80.0	66.7	80.0	50.0	66.7	50.0
4. College — varied courses	—	—	—	12.5	33.3	50.0
5. College — 2-year degree	—	—	—	—	—	—
6. College — 4-year degree	60.0	—	—	—	—	—
7. 3-year diploma school	—	—	—	—	—	—
8. 12-month LPN school	—	—	—	—	—	—
9. 18-month LPN school	—	33.3	—	—	—	—
10. College-based training	20.0	—	—	—	—	—
11. Hospital-based training	20.0	—	—	—	—	—
12. Depends on individual	—	—	—	25.0	—	—
Total number of individuals interviewed	5	3	5	8	3	8

Source: *Utilization of Health Personnel: A Five Hospital Study,* appendix, table VII-18, p. A243.

[1]May not add to 100 percent because more than one answer was given in some cases.

Cressyda

Table 37. Percentage Distribution of Allied Health Personnel by Extent to Which the Following Experiences Prepared Them for the Function They Are Presently Performing[1]

Extent to which the following prepared them for their present function	General Nursing RN	LPN	Senior nursing technician	Nursing technician	Senior nursing assistant	Nursing assistant
High school	8.0	—	7.0	63.5	13.3	16.2
College	10.0	—	—	—	—	—
Vocational/technical training	—	—	1.0	—	—	—
On-the-job training	21.0	30.0	32.0	52.7	37.8	39.4
Professional training	32.0	38.3	25.0	10.0	—	5.6
Practical experiences	29.0	31.7	35.0	31.0	48.9	38.8
Other	—	—	—	—	—	—
Total number of individuals interviewed	5	3	5	8	3	8

Source: *Utilization of Health Personnel: A Five Hospital Study*, appendix, table A88, p. A246.

[1]May not add to 100 percent because of rounding.

Cressyda

Table 38. Percentage Distribution of Allied Health Personnel by the Occupational Level They Can Realistically Hope to Attain with Their Present Educational and Professional Training[1]

Occupational level they can realistically hope to attain	RN	LPN	Senior nursing technician	Nursing technician	Senior nursing assistant	Nursing assistant
Can go higher and would like to	20.0	33.3	20.0	12.5	66.7	25.0
Can go higher, but would not like to	—	—	—	—	—	—
Can go higher, but unclear if respondent would like to or not	80.0	—	—	62.5	33.3	75.0
Total: Can go higher	100.0	33.3	20.0	75.0	100.0	100.0
Dead end, but would like to go higher	—	—	—	25.0	—	—
Dead end, but satisfied	—	33.3	—	—	—	—
Dead end, but unclear if respondent is satisfied or not	—	33.3	60.0	—	—	—
Total: Dead end	—	66.6	60.0	25.0	—	—
Would have to leave hospital to go higher and might consider it	—	—	—	—	—	—
Would have to leave hospital to go higher but don't intend to	—	—	—	—	—	—
Total: Must leave to advance	—	—	—	—	—	—
Generally unsure	—	—	20.0	—	—	—
Total number of individuals interviewed	5	3	5	8	3	8

Source: *Utilization of Health Personnel: A Five Hospital Study*, Vol. 2, table A87, p. A245.

[1] May not add to 100 percent because of rounding or because more than one answer was given.

Cressyda

Table 39. Percentage Distribution of Allied Health Personnel by Their Plans for Future Employment and Their Reasons[1]

Future plans and reasons for them	RN	LPN	Senior nursing technician	Nursing technician	Senior nursing assistant	Nursing assistant
Plan to remain at this hospital	100.0	33.3	100.0	62.5	100.0	37.5
Plan to leave	—	33.3	—	12.5	—	50.0
Plan to stay indefinitely	—	33.3	—	—	—	—
No plans/unsure	—	—	—	25.0	—	12.5
Reasons for remaining:						
1. Like the work/people	40.0	—	60.0	12.5	66.7	12.5
2. Convenience	—	—	20.0	—	—	—
3. Settled here	—	—	—	—	—	—
4. Employee/retirement benefits	—	—	20.0	—	—	—
5. Good salary	—	—	—	—	—	—
6. No place else to go	—	—	—	—	—	—
7. Other/none	60.0	66.7	—	50.0	33.3	25.0
Reasons for leaving:						
1. Personal reasons	—	33.3	—	12.5	—	12.5
2. Temporary employment	—	—	—	—	—	—
3. Dissatisfied with working conditions	—	—	—	—	—	12.5
4. Cannot advance here	—	—	—	—	—	—
5. Returning to school	—	—	—	—	—	37.5
6. Completion of alternative service (C.O.)	—	—	—	—	—	—
7. Other/none	—	—	—	—	—	—
Total number of individuals interviewed	5	3	5	8	3	8

Source: *Utilization of Health Personnel: A Five Hospital Study*, Vol. 2, table VII-21, p. A247.

[1] May not add to 100 percent because of rounding or because more than one answer was given.

8

Guide for Restructuring Health Occupations

We have indicated how the utilization of allied health personnel in a number of hospitals was analyzed and have presented a summary of the findings. In these hospitals, a consistent pattern of manpower utilization emerged, characterized by considerable overlap of functions by related professions; little in-service training; little possibility of upgrading or promotion from within; and hiring standards placed at a level unnecessarily high for achieving effective job performance and for obtaining a ready supply of labor.

Manpower Utilization Survey

Because our findings and conclusions were based on a research project in five diverse hospitals, one could question whether the findings are applicable to any single health provider. To undertake the restructuring of an occupational hierarchy when it is not necessary would be wasteful. If a hospital is utilizing its health personnel efficiently, there is no need to restructure occupations; our findings are not applicable. However, we must conclude from our findings that most hospitals are not operating at or near 100 percent efficient utilization of their health personnel. If a hospital is uncertain and prefers to conduct its own investigation, it can be done, in a summary fashion, as follows:

1. Select one or more departments for investigation. Depending on the size and type of hospital, one may analyze only one department, such as general nursing service, or one may include others, such as the x-ray department and the laboratory. Someone from the staff should be assigned as project director, with prime responsibility for all aspects of the research.

2. Explain, in detail, to all personnel and to any unions in the department involved, the purpose of the investigation. To gain the cooperation of all personnel, assurances must be given that no employees will be disadvantaged by the study.

3. Using the appropriate list of functions and the appropriate questionnaire, interview a sample of employees in the department.[1] To assure the employees of a measure of confidentiality, it is preferable that the interviewer be someone from outside the hospital or a nonsupervisor from some other department.

4. Analyze the responses. Determine whether the hiring-in qualifications are relevant to the performance of functions on which the employees spend a major share of their time. Determine whether there is substantial overlap of functions being performed by persons in different occupations. Determine whether a significant portion of the functions performed by persons in a specific occupation is below the level of skill normally expected of that occupation.

5. Based on the findings, decide whether or not the employees are being utilized efficiently. If the findings indicate substantial inefficiencies, the situation then warrants some effort to restructure the occupational hierarchy and to make other changes that improve the utilization of health personnel.

Some Survey Techniques

In the following discussion we describe the methodology used to arrive at our conclusions on the current utilization of health manpower in hospitals. Included are guidelines and instructions on conducting a survey of health personnel in a single facility, as well as criteria for comparing the results with the results of our research efforts. We also have included explanations on how to use the questionnaire, how to tabulate and interpret the results, as well as how to determine where the utilization of health workers could be improved.

Questionnaires and the Interview Process

Before undertaking the actual investigation of what is being done by whom in a specific department, it is important that a detailed questionnaire be developed and tested. (See end of this chapter for a sample questionnaire.) When this has been completed, the interviewers should become familiar with the questionnaire, the occupations and the task definitions[2] and should be trained in the techniques of interviewing. At an early stage of the undertaking, all personnel in departments that are to be analyzed should be informed of what is to be done, and the purpose of the undertaking should be carefully explained to them. In reference to the questionnaire, each respondent should be assured that the information given in the interviews will be confidential and that no names will be associated with individual responses.

The first part of the questionnaire should include all questions relating to background and personal attributes. The second part of the interview should cover the functions that may be performed by the occupation in question. The basic purpose of this part of the questionnaire is to determine the amount of time spent on a series of functions, which is transformed into a percentage of the work-week spent on each function. (See end of this chapter, where a sample interview is entered on questionnaire and the information is tabulated in such a way that summary tables can be constructed.)

Construction of Summary Tables

The direct data from the questionnaire provide information that must be synthesized in summary form. The following procedure was used to arrive at the summary table for each occupation:

1. Each questionnaire was evaluated and the percentage of time spent on each function was reduced proportionately so that the total equaled 100 percent. To accomplish this, the percentage of time spent on all functions was totalled and then divided into 100. The result was a reducing factor that decreased the given percents to actual percentage, totalling 100 percent. These are the adjusted percentages of time spent on each function. It was assumed that there was no distortion in the relative importance of each function, only in the number assigned to it.

2. Using these adjusted percentages of time for each person interviewed, all the percentages for all those interviewed were totalled for each specific function. (See end of chapter for sample worksheet.)

3. Each of these totals was multiplied by 2,400 (minutes in an average workweek) to get the total number of minutes spent on each function by those who perform it.

4. The number of minutes spent on each function was totalled for all functions and then a percentage distribution for each function was calculated.

Guidelines for Restructuring Manpower

In this project, which involved the restructuring of functions of health personnel in five hospitals, we were relatively successful. However, we had had the benefit of considerable experience in techniques of restructuring occupational hierarchies in The Cambridge Hospital, and our years of work on these problems may partially account for our success. Another factor may have been that, although we were working with widely diverse hospitals, a sample of five in the New England area may not be representative of hospitals in the rest of the United States. While the five hospital study confirmed our methodolgies for analyzing the occupational structures and for restructuring the occupations, the critical test will be whether these experiments can be replicated in different hospitals across the nation.

There is no surefire set of steps that guarantees success in any effort to restructure the allied health occupations of a hospital. Based on our experience, we offer the following as important guidelines:

1. At the outset and throughout the program, it is imperative that the administrator be thoroughly convinced of the importance of the effort. Support for the program must be demonstrated enthusiastically and must be reinforced constantly. Some changes will not come easily or will come very slowly, and unless the administrator is completely convinced of the value of the changes, efforts may waver and ultimately fail.

2. An initial step is the formation of a committee on restructuring. This committee should include the director of nursing, heads of departments to be affected, as well as representatives from all segments of the hospital community. Such a composition will facilitate communications and help increase the cooperation of all concerned. This committee should be charged with the major tasks of analyzing the job functions of all health care occupations and of recommending all changes needed to improve the utilization of personnel.

3. The committee must then adopt a job description and a list of important functions for each major health care occupation.

4. Where there is significant or substantial overlap of functions, the committee should recommend a shifting of functions so that the more sophisticated or complex functions will be performed by the higher-skilled occupations, and the less sophisticated or simple tasks will be performed by the lower-skilled occupations. This should improve the utilization of manpower and also improve the quality of service in the hospital. Great care must be taken in introducing changes in this sensitive area, and employees affected must be given assurances that their earnings and job security will not be affected negatively.

5. In addition to analyzing job functions for each occupation, the restructuring committee should examine the hiring-in requirements as they relate to job descriptions and functions. For example, is it necessary for aides or ward clerks to have high school diplomas? Are the hiring standards arbitrarily screening out entry-level personnel from among disadvantaged and minor-

ity groups? Where a labor shortage exists, in-service programs should be provided to bring entry-level personnel up to desired competence levels in basic skills.

6. If the attrition rate is high, it may be because of lack of in-service training and of opportunities for upward mobility of employees. Under these conditions, it would be important to establish an in-service education department, either by setting up training programs within the hospital or by hiring specialists to conduct classroom education and supervise on-the-job training. Although in-service educational programs are costly, our findings indicate that in the long run such programs more than pay for themselves in the form of a reduced attrition rate and increased job satisfaction.

7. Programs that permit or encourage upward mobility offer tremendous job satisfaction to the employees involved, as well as the opportunity for job advancement and higher earnings, and should be incorporated in any occupational restructuring plans. One such in-service training program involves a progression of advancement from nursing assistant trainee to senior nursing assistant to nursing technician to senior nursing technician. The training course for nursing assistant is offered to persons with no previous training; the course is brief and is divided equally. between supervised work and didactic training. Advancement to the next higher occupation is usually based on evidence of proficiency as observed by the individual's supervisor. In one hospital a successful program of career ladders allows entry-level personnel to move up through the ranks in several areas, including nursing, clerical, and laboratory. The program allows LPNs to receive registered nursing degrees through a two-year program which accepts their previous LPN experience toward a more advanced degree.

8. Because of relatively rapid changes in technology, equipment, and hospital policy, it is important to offer all health personnel continuing in-service education programs. All personnel should be encouraged to register for such courses. If such programs are not feasible, another way of encouraging further training is for the hospital to arrange for a program of reimbursement of tuition and book costs at an educational institution.

9. An important adjunct to job restructuring, in-service train-

ing, and upward job mobility is compensation appropriate to the duties of the job. New titles and new responsibilities are important to job satisfaction, but a salary adjustment is generally critical if there is to be long-term interest in the position. There should be distinct differentials in salaries between steps on the job ladder. In general, our experiences indicate that the increases in compensation will be offset by the improvement in personnel utilization, the increase in job satisfaction, and the decline in absenteeism, tardiness, and turnover.

10. Some of the most creative innovations have been introduced by ideas and suggestions made by employees at all levels. Such employee participation should be encouraged.

11. For a program, whatever its scope, to be successful, the administrator must use whatever resources are available to assure all personnel, trustees, and unions within the facility that an effective restructuring will benefit the total institution and improve the quality of care, that while most individuals and groups will gain, none will lose.

We believe we have demonstrated that it is advantageous for hospitals to institute career ladders and in-service training. Our research findings indicate that the present lack of vertical mobility is inefficient and wasteful in the use of health care personnel. To what degree the overlapping of job functions should be tolerated varies with the situation in individual facilities. In the face of rising costs and increased demand, the health care delivery system will be forced to adapt. However, there is no one set of standards to determine an unacceptable degree of overlap. A hospital evaluating the utilization of its personnel must examine its priorities. Does the outcome of the survey single out any areas that are ripe for restructuring? Where can employees and patients benefit from a reassigning of particular tasks? Are hiring standards for any particular occupation higher or lower than necessary to perform the job?

It would be ludicrous to suggest that physicians, registered nurses, or any other of the many health occupations should perform only the most sophisticated functions for which they were trained. For example, registered nurses cannot be expected to perform at their most sophisticated level forty hours a week, fifty weeks a year. This is obviously true for any occupation. However, in light of rising health costs and the increasing demand for health services, it is difficult to justify the opposite extreme.

If a hospital finds that all its registered nurses are spending 30 percent of their time on group 1 functions (the simplest functions) and aides are spending an equal percentage of their time on group 3 functions, something is clearly wrong. The situation is even worse if the hospital is fully aware that its aides have not received proper in-service education or on-the-job training programs qualifying them to perform the more sophisticated functions.

A hospital should examine closely those health occupations that experience high turnover rates and persistent vacancies. It is in these occupations that the hospital may receive fairly rapid compensation in terms of lower turnover rates and increased job satisfaction by instituting realistic job ladders, in-service training and job restructuring.

Interview Sample

BACKGROUND INFORMATION

1. Name: _____Susan Jones_____

2. Job Title: _____Registered Nurse_____

3. Age: _____36_____ 4. Sex: _____F_____

5. Education:

	No. of Years	Name of School or Hospital	Degree Completed
Grammar School	8		
High School	4		yes
College	1	U. of Mass	no

6. Additional Professional Training (explain): ____3-year diploma school____

_____

7. On-the-Job Training (explain): _Yes. 1 day-course on EKG machine___ operation after working here for several years. Would like more.

_____

8. Professional Certification (specify): _____R.N._____

_____

9. Are you a student at present? _____No_____

Name of Program   Institution

_____   _____

Date Started   Completion Date

_____   _____

10. Do you receive a stipend or other form of financial support? ___No____

_____

11. Do you pay tuition? (specify) _____No_____

_____

12. How long have you been employed at your present profession? _____ 14 years

_____

    a. At this hospital? _____ 12 years _____

    b. Elsewhere? (specify) __ 1 year, City Hospital & 1 year, __

    _____ Metropolitan State Hospital _____

    c. If elsewhere, how or why did you come to _____

    Hospital? _____ More benefits, better pay, closer to home _____

    _____

13. Have you been employed at any other health-related occupation? __ No __

    _____

    Specify: _____

    When: _____

    Where: _____

    How long: _____

14. Exactly how detailed was your orientation after accepting your present job?
    _____ Not detailed at all _____

    a. Length of orientation: _____ 1 day _____

    b. Class work involved: _ 1 hr. orientation to hospital policies _

    c. Other: _____ Head nurse explained duties on the floor _____

15. Exactly how would you train or orient a new employee in your field?

    a. On-the-Job: _____ 2-week on-the-job program _____

    b. Classes in hospital: _ At least 1 hr. a day along with on-the-job training _

    _____

    c. Other: _____ It is important to become familiar with other _____

    departments, know where to find answers to questions.

16. What formal level of education should be required in your field? _____
    3-year diploma school is sufficient for the RN's job as it is here.

    _____

17. What personal qualities should be required in your department or field?
    Patience, stamina, professional attitudes toward patients and their problems.

18. What occupational level can you realistically hope to attain with your present educational and professional training? (Explain fully) Up some existing occupational ladder? Dead-end? If dead-end, why?

   Here, can't advance without a B.S. Degree

19. To what extent did exposure to the following prepare you for the function you are presently performing?   Percent

   High School ———————————————————————— —

   College ——————————————————————————— 25%

   Vocational/Technical Training —————————————— —

   On-the-Job Training —————————————————————— —

   Professional Training ——————————————————— 50%

   Practical Experiences —————————————————— 25%

   Other —————————————————————————————— —

20. Do you expect to remain at this hospital? Why or why not?
   Yes, this is a good environment, a progressive teaching hospital

21. General Comments: She feels frustrated, can't go further here— would like to do more sophisticated tasks than she is allowed.

I. Name: _____ Susan Jones _____

II. Job Title: _____ Registered Nurse _____

III. Department: _____ GENERAL NURSING SERVICE _____

Which of the following functions are you presently performing?	Yes or No	Not Done This Department	Percentage of Time Spent on Each Function	Reducing Factor $100 \div 255$	Adjusted Percentage of Time Spent on Each Function
1. Straightening up and cleaning: patients' immediate furniture, nurses station, utility rooms, treatment rooms, nourishment center, and litters	yes		13	.4	5.1
2. Distributing mail and flowers	no		—	.4	0
3. Doing department errands: going to orthopedic department, Central Supply, laundry, IBM or records office, or operating room to help bring back a patient	yes		8	.4	3.1
4. Doing errands for patient: making phone calls, refilling water jugs, preparing snacks or drinks from nourishment station, getting an extra pillow	yes		25	.4	9.8
5. Giving and removing bedpans, assisting patient to use bedpan or urinal, helping patient to and from bathroom	yes		8	.4	3.1
6. Making beds: unoccupied, occupied, post-operative	yes		5	.4	2.0
7. Answering patient calls	yes		5	.4	2.0

Item				
8. Admitting patient: completing clothes list or valuables list, getting patient settled in bed, notifying intern	yes	3	.4	1.2
9. Discharging patient: returning clothes and valuables, accompanying patient from floor	yes	3	.4	1.2
10. Locating and setting up simple equipment: bed rails, footboards, sandbags, heel coverlets	yes	8	.4	3.1
11. Taking patient to x-ray; taking lab specimens to lab	yes	8	.4	3.1
12. Assisting in moving patients to another floor	yes	1	.4	.4
13. Measuring food and fluid intake and output and totaling: urine jugs, tube drainage, and IV intake at the end of each shift	yes	8	.4	3.1
14. Checking, delivering, and picking up food trays; feeding patients	yes	8	.4	3.1
15. Putting away supplies, instruments, and equipment	yes	1	.4	.4
16. Washing or soaking used equipment and supplies, putting them on the cart to be returned to Central Supply	yes	1	.4	.4
17. Caring for deceased persons	yes	1	.4	.4
18. Giving information or directions to patients or visitors, or directing them to the correct source of information	yes	3	.4	1.2
19. Collecting urine, stool, or sputum specimens to be sent to lab; performing routine tests; obtaining a culture	yes	8	.4	3.1
20. Giving routine morning care	yes	21	.4	8.2
21. Preparing patients for bed at night	yes	8	.4	3.1
22. Assisting patients with walkers, wheelchairs, crutches, and braces	yes	3	.4	1.2
23. Lifting patients on and off litters	yes	1	.4	.4

(continued)

24. Taking and recording: temperature, pulse, respiration rate, blood pressure, and weight	yes	8	.4	3.1
25. Assisting patient with sitz bath	yes	1	.4	.4
26. Applying or changing: ice bags, hot water bottles, ace bandages, elastic stockings, binders, slings, restraints	yes	8	.4	3.1
27. Giving cleansing treatments: enemas, douches	yes	3	.4	1.2
28. Caring for wounds: dressing, irrigating, changing dressings	yes	13	.4	5.1
29. Feeding patient by tube	yes	3	.4	1.2
30. Caring for precaution or reverse precaution patients	yes	1	.4	.4
31. Setting up suture sets, assisting doctor in removing sutures	Removes sutures herself / yes	1	.4	.4
32. Doing cervical smears; venereal disease smears	yes	1	.4	.4
33. Assisting doctor in wart removal; skin biopsies	no	0	.4	0
34. Washing and dressing lacerations	yes	1	.4	.4
35. Using EKG equipment		0	.4	0
36. Drawing blood	yes	1	.4	.4
37. Ordering drugs from pharmacy; receiving and putting away drugs		1	.4	.4
38. Administering specified medication; noting time and amounts on patients' charts	yes	1	.4	.4
39. Performing functions related to oxygen masks and catheters	yes	15	.4	5.9
40. Performing functions relating to IV's	yes	1	.4	.4
41. Assisting physicians during treatment and examination of patients	yes	3	.4	1.2
42. Counting narcotics and barbiturates at the change of each shift	yes	3	.4	1.2

Item				
43. Observing and reporting to supervisor or physician on patient's condition, reaction to drugs, treatments, I.V.s, significant incidents	yes	3	.4	1.2
44. Serving emotional support to patients; entertaining patients (particularly children)	yes	3	.4	1.2
45. Participating in cardiac arrest team	yes	1	.4	.4
46. Beginning preparations for patient scheduled for surgery	yes	2	.4	.8
47. Filling out accident reports	yes	1	.4	.4
48. Stamping lab slips and requisitions, making necessary arrangements for x-rays and lab work	yes	3	.4	1.2
49. Checking and posting orders in MD order books	yes	3	.4	1.2
50. Checking off diet manual each shift	yes	1	.4	.4
51. Recommending or arranging for a consultation with medical specialists, social services, psychiatry, etc.	yes	1	.4	.4
52. Assigning and coordinating nursing activities, including making out daily assignment sheet	yes	3	.4	1.2
53. Evaluating quality of nursing care	yes	1	.4	.4
54. Observing nursing care and visiting patients regularly to ensure proper nursing care	yes	1	.4	.4
55. Regularly inspecting rooms and wards for cleanliness and comfort	yes	1	.4	.4
56. Accompanying physicians on rounds	yes	3	.4	1.2
57. Investigating and adjusting complaints	yes	1	.4	.4
58. Supervising preparation and maintenance of patients' clinical records	no	1	.4	.4
59. Giving change-of-shift report	yes	5	.4	2.0
60. Teaching	yes	3	.4	1.2
61. Research				
62. Supervisory duties	yes	1	.4	.4

(continued)

no

63. Waiting for work
64. Caring for mother in labor
65. Assisting in delivery room
66. Caring for newborn
67. Caring for mother after delivery
68. Preparing babies or children for afternoon
naps, including bathing, diapering, giving
bottle, if applicable

Total % of time spent on all functions = 255%
Reducing Factor Total to 100% = 100 ÷ 255 = .4

WORKSHEET SAMPLE

	Interview 1	Interview 2	Interview 3	Interview 4	Total % of Time Spent by 1-2-3-4	Column A X 2400
					A	B
1	5.1	1.1	6.2	1.4	13.8	33120
2	0	0	.3	0	.3	720
3	3.1	0	0	.5	3.6	8640
4	9.8	1.1	.3	.5	11.7	28080
5	3.1	8.0	7.4	3.8	22.3	53520
6	2.0	8.0	6.2	1.4	17.6	42480
7	2.0	8.0	.9	3.8	14.7	35280
8	1.2	3.0	6.2	1.4	11.8	28320
9	1.2	1.1	2.4	.5	5.2	12480
10	3.1	4.9	.3	.5	8.8	21120
11	3.1	0	0	0	3.1	7440
12	.4	.4	.9	.5	2.2	5280
13	3.1	4.9	.3	1.4	9.7	23280
14	3.1	4.9	7.4	3.8	19.2	46080
15	.4	0	.9	.5	1.8	4320
16	.4	0	0	0	.4	960
17	.4	.4	.3	.5	1.6	3840
18	1.2	1.1	.3	.5	3.1	7440
				Group 1 Total Minutes —	362400	
19	3.1	1.1	.9	.5	5.6	13440
20	8.2	9.8	7.4	12.0	37.4	98760
21	3.1	.4	7.4	.5	11.4	27360
22	1.2	3.0	0	1.4	5.6	13440
23	.4	1.1	.9	.5	2.9	6960
24	3.1	4.9	.9	1.4	10.3	24720
25	.4	.4	.3	.5	1.6	3840
26	3.1	3.0	.9	1.4	8.4	20160
27	1.2	1.1	.9	.5	3.7	8880
28	5.1	3.0	.9	1.4	10.4	24960
29	1.2	.4	2.4	.5	4.5	10800
30	.4	.4	.3	1.4	2.5	6000
				Group 2 Total Minutes —	259320	
31	.4	0	.3	.5	1.2	2880
32	0	0	0	.5	.5	1200
33	.4	0	.3	0	.7	1680
34	0	0	.3	.5	.8	1920
35	.4	0	0	0	.4	960

(continued)

(continued)

36	.4	0	0	0	.4	960
37	.4	0	.9	.5	1.8	4320
38	5.9	1.1	7.4	12.0	26.4	63360
39	.4	1.1	.9	1.4	3.8	9120
40	—	—	—	—	—	—
41	1.2	3.0	2.4	3.8	10.4	24960
42	1.2	1.1	2.4	1.4	6.1	14640
43	.4	.4	.9	.5	2.2	5280
44	1.2	1.9	.9	1.4	5.4	12960
45	1.2	3.0	2.4	1.4	8.0	19200
46	.4	0	.9	0	1.3	3120
47	.8	3.0	.3	.5	4.6	11040

Group 3 Total Minutes — 177600

48	.4	.4	.9	.5	2.2	5280
49	1.2	.4	.3	1.4	3.3	7920
50	1.2	.4	2.4	1.4	5.4	12960
51	.4	.4	.9	.5	2.2	5280
52	.4	0	.9	.5	1.8	4320
53	1.2	0	.9	.5	2.6	6240
54	.4	0	0	1.4	1.8	4320
55	.4	1.1	2.4	3.8	7.7	18420
56	.4	0	.3	.5	1.2	2880
57	1.2	.4	2.4	0	4.0	9600
58	.4	1.1	.9	.5	2.9	6960
59	.4	1.1	0	0	1.5	3600
60	2.0	1.1	.9	1.4	5.4	12960
61	1.2	1.1	2.4	3.8	8.5	20400
62	0	0	0	0	0	0
63	.4	0	0	10.1	10.5	25200

Group 4 Total Minutes — 142500

64	0	.4	0	1.4	1.8	4320
65	0	0	0	0	0	0
66	0	0	0	0	0	0
67	0	0	0	0	0	0
68	0	0	0	0	0	0
69	0	0	0	0	0	0

Group 5 Total Minutes — 4320

Totals by Group	Column B	% by Group
Group 1	362400	38.3
Group 2	259320	27.4
Group 3	177600	18.8
Group 4	142500	15.1
Group 5	4320	.4
Grand Total = 946140		100.0

9

Summary and Conclusions

Over the past decade, the Center for Medical Manpower Studies of the Department of Economics of Northeastern University has been involved in a series of research projects concerned with the utilization of health care personnel, especially in hospitals. We proceeded from a pilot study to an in-depth single hospital study and demonstration project to the five hospital study described in this volume. The findings in these studies were cumulative and corroborative.

The hypothesis of the pilot study, our initial work in the area of health care personnel, was that hiring-in standards for health personnel in hospitals are higher than necessary. The findings of that study substantiate the hypothesis. Although the hiring standards in hospitals are generally established either on a departmental or general administrative basis, the accrediting agencies and professional societies have considerable influence over hiring-in requirements for a number of health occupations. These agencies and societies have a vested interest in maintaining high education and training standards, and the result has been high-level requirements for most occupations, even those at the entry-level position. Similarly, educational institutions also have a strong interest in maintaining or raising the educational and training requirements to enter health care occupations as health training programs are being offered by a growing number of educational institutions. Even the most unskilled health occupations in hospitals frequently require a high school diploma.

Our pilot study showed that when a situation was critical, hospitals did hire persons without a high school education and such persons did perform as well as those with the high school diploma. The high school requirement was often retained despite numbers of individuals without the diploma being hired. Retaining such a standard made it very difficult for educationally deprived persons (especially among ethnic and racial minorities) to obtain health care jobs in hospitals even when labor shortages existed.

Although the pilot study focused on hiring standards, it also produced some evidence that health personnel in entry-level positions, without prior education or training, did perform rather sophisticated and high-level functions. In addition, there was some evidence that persons in high-level positions that required years of education and training spent substantial amounts of time on very simple functions. There was no doubt that an overlap of functions existed; what was not known was the extent and the degree.

In our follow-up study, an in-depth analysis of the utilization of health manpower was done in a single institution, The Cambridge Hospital. After months of observing health care personnel in numerous occupations performing various tasks and functions and of interviewing a sample of persons in the different health occupations, the hypothesis of the original study was again confirmed. The hiring-in standards were higher than necessary and there was considerable overlap of functions.

An analysis of the data and information obtained at The Cambridge Hospital showed that a substantial proportion of entry-level personnel performed many of the highly sophisticated and complex tasks and that the time they spent on these functions was not trivial. At the same time, personnel in the high-level positions did perform many of the simple functions and spent a substantial proportion of their time on these functions.

In this in-depth single hospital study, we also studied a whole range of personnel practices, along with such employment factors as on-the-job training, attrition, and job satisfaction. Our findings were not novel, but they confirmed the general impression that the health care industry, particularly the hospitals, provided employment largely in dead-end jobs, with little job satisfaction and relatively little opportunity for training and for upward job mobility. In many instances professional organizations imposed entrance barriers by requiring years of education and training at educational institutions; experience and training on the job were not considered as substitutes for formal education.

As a result of these findings, we recommended to The Cambridge Hospital a series of changes aimed at improving the hospital's utilization of health care personnel. Over a relatively short period of time, the hospital adopted many of the recommendations. The hiring-in requirements were lowered, thereby making high school dropouts eligible for employment in a number of entry-level occupations. A number of training programs were started, thereby permitting employees to keep current in a rapidly changing environment and making some upward mobility possible. These changes had some impact on improving job satisfaction. Job functions and duties were redefined to some extent, eliminating some overlap, and making it possible to establish new classifications with new duties and functions. Overall, there were substantial improvements in the utilization of health personnel.

As these personnel changes were being made in the hospital, a number of other changes were occurring, some of which were directly related to the personnel changes, while others cannot be readily associated with them. The hospital occupancy rate increased; the mortality and morbidity rates declined; hospital costs decreased. At a minimum, one can conclude that the quality of service to hospital patients did not decline and perhaps increased slightly.

It was important to know that one could obtain the cooperation of a hospital in analyzing the utilization of its health care personnel and in making changes to improve the utilization. However, there was no certainty that the cooperation of The Cambridge Hospital and the results of our joint efforts were not unique. It became important to determine whether other types of hospitals would be willing to analyze the utilization of their personnel and whether the results in other hospitals would be substantially the same as in The Cambridge Hospital.

In the five hospital study we obtained the cooperation of five basically different types of hospitals. The results of our study in these hospitals largely substantiate our earlier findings on the utilization of health care personnel.

The findings described in chapter 6 demonstrated the overlap of functions among workers of different skill levels. A large proportion of medical functions are performed by all types of nursing personnel from RNs to nurse's aides. The assignment of what are considered the most difficult nursing tasks to lesser-skilled workers seems to be a very common practice. Its prevalence suggests that lower-level nursing personnel perform these tasks very effectively. On the other hand, RNs spend considerable time performing the least difficult nursing tasks. The distribution of the nursing personnel's time over tasks of varying complexity indicates that the informal organization of work on the ward does not necessarily coincide with the formal hierarchy.

There are undoubtedly many reasons for this, but in a recent article D.C. Feldman argued that the nurse's role, in particular, is full of conflicts. Feldman found that, of all the occupational groups he surveyed in a 350-bed community hospital, nurses had the most difficulty in role definition and in agreeing with supervisors on work evaluation. There was a noticeable discrepancy between how three-year diploma nurses and four-year degree nurses defined their roles. The three-year nurses tended to think that keeping on schedule, handling all patients efficiently, and being responsive to the requests of doctors were the marks of a good nurse. The four-year nurses wished to focus on total patient care and felt they should share in diagnosis and treatment decisions. These two views of nursing involve different task priorities, and head nurses varied in how they expected their staff to perform. Conflicting expectations fostered a very low level of general satisfaction among the nurses in that study.[1]

It seems reasonable to assume that the overlap in functions we have documented in this study is partly the result of conflicting expectations and inadequately defined job responsibilities. Although personnel at different skill levels may perform a wide range of tasks in a satisfactory manner, incongruence between expectations, training, and task assignments can lead to low morale among workers.

In theory, one way to minimize job dissatisfaction is to orient workers to their jobs so that their expectations are congruent with the actual demands of the job. With the exception of Cressyda, the hospitals in the study gave most of their workers relatively short orientations, which often consisted of nothing more than an introduction to hospital policies. Although most of the persons interviewed thought the orientation they received was appropriate, it is questionable whether hospital orientation programs actually accomplish what administrators and supervisors expect of them. The supervisors in Feldman's study thought that orientation sessions improved the workers' morale, but his analysis showed that neither motivation nor involvement in one's work were influenced by the initial "socialization" period. Feldman concludes: "Managers may need to look more to the design of individual jobs and work groups to increase the motivation and job involvement of employees, and to special training interventions to improve communication."[2]

The task of providing constant care to seriously ill people creates its own kind of organizational problems. When a task needs to be done on a hospital ward, particularly in an emergency or when the floor is understaffed, anyone who is available helps where he or she is needed. Consequently, the informal organization of workers that occurs in the actual performance of patient care tasks may not follow the formal personnel hierarchy. Although responsibilities constantly overlap, "lower-skilled," lower-paid personnel are not officially given credit for performing the more demanding tasks which they often find themselves doing. The lack of a realistic job ladder by which employees who have mastered new skills can move into better-paying jobs adds to the general dissatisfaction.

In general, we found that, with minor, marginal differences, each of the five hospitals included in the study had significant weaknesses in the utilization of its health care personnel. The most common defects in personnel utilization were:

1. Substantial overlap of functions
2. Little or no on-the-job training for advancement
3. Little or no on-the-job training to keep current in one's profession
4. Dead-end nature of most entry-level positions

5. Low job satisfaction, especially among personnel in entry-level positions

6. High turnover rates, with concomitant high personnel costs

The following general conclusions can be drawn from this research:

1. Five diverse hospitals in the New England area were willing to cooperate in our study and to have their occupational structure and related personnel practices analyzed.

2. Despite the diversity of the five hospitals, it was found that in each of the hospitals health care employees with less than the specified required experience and training were competently performing functions of a difficult nature, not commonly associated with entry-level occupations.

3. Health personnel with more sophisticated training and experience (for example, physicians, RNs, and technologists) were found to be underutilized, that is, spending a significant amount of their time performing simple medical functions. A reorganization of their medical functions (eliminating them from the "easy" tasks by substituting other classifications of adequately trained health personnel) could lead to a more efficient utilization of their training and experience.

4. The efforts made by some hospitals in the area of restructuring health occupations has led to greater job satisfaction and consequently to lower turnover rates and the reduction of dead-end, entry-level positions.

5. Specific measures of acceptable professional task performance have yet to be developed for most categories of health personnel. Without such standards, those involved in occupational restructuring efforts are open to criticism on the grounds that quality is being sacrificed for the sake of cost containment.

6. Despite the various changes in personnel policies and practices made by these hospitals, it appears that the quality of service to the patients has not declined and actually may have risen.

7 If the five hospitals studied were willing to undergo an analysis of their health personnel and to make some changes that improved the utilization of their personnel, then it is likely that many other hospitals across the nation are prepared to undergo a similar analysis.

8. The procedures and techniques for analyzing the utilization of health personnel are not so arcane that they cannot be reproduced by hospital administrators after relatively little study.

9. Once a hospital has analyzed the utilization of its personnel, it is likely to introduce some changes that will improve that utilization.

10. Continued publicity on the benefits of analyzing the utilization of health personnel and of reorganizing occupational structure and functions is likely to entice more and more hospitals to undertake some aspects of restructuring their health care occupations.

11. Health providers, especially hospitals and educational institutions that specialize in training health personnel, must be encouraged to establish academic integrity in their various programs. Far too often they are convinced by professional health personnel associations that degree-granting programs are necessary for the establishment and maintenance of professional standards of practice. In their attempts to persuade, professional associations are motivated by the wish to legitimate the positions of their professions within the health care system. When such efforts merely lead to the erection of employment barriers, especially barriers against entry-level personnel, they should be discouraged by hospitals and educational institutions.

12. When some form of national health insurance is passed by Congress, there will be a substantial increase in the demand for health care personnel. The anticipated shortage in those health care professions that require long-term education and training could be reduced by widespread restructuring of the health care occupations in hospitals.

Notes

CHAPTER 1

1. Executive Office of the President, Council on Wages and Price Stability, *The Problem of Rising Health Care Costs,* Staff Report (Washington, D.C.: Government Printing Office, April 1976), pp. 1-3.

2. American Hospital Association, *Hospital Statistics* (Chicago: American Hospital Association, 1977), pp. 2-3.

3. University of Michigan School of Public Health, *The Report of the Commission on Education for Health Administraton,* Vol. 1 (Ann Arbor, Mich.: Health Administration Press, 1975), p. 16.

CHAPTER 2

1. Walter Franke and Irvin Sobel, *The Shortage of Skilled and Technical Workers* (Lexington, Mass.: D.C. Heath and Co., Lexington Books, 1970), pp. 70-71.

2. U.S. Department of Labor, Bureau of Labor Statistics, *Annual Earnings and Employment Patterns of Private Nonagricultural Employees, 1965,* Bulletin 1675 (Washington, D.C.: Government Printing Office, 1971), table 1, pp. 9-10.

3. U.S. Department of Labor, Bureau of Labor Statistics, *Industry and Wage Survey, Hospitals, March 1969,* Bulletin 1688 (Washington, D.C.: Government Printing Office, 1971), pp. 14-15.

4. Harry I. Greenfield, *Allied Health Manpower: Trends and Prospects* (New York: Columbia University Press, 1969), p. vii.

5. Eli Ginzberg and Miriam Ostow, *Men, Money, and Medicine* (New York: Columbia University Press, 1969), p. 153.

6. Morris A. Horowitz and Harold M. Goldstein, *Hiring Standards for Paramedical Manpower* (Boston: Center for Medical Manpower Studies (CMMS),

Northeastern University, 1968, under grant from the U.S. Department of Labor, Manpower Administration). This study is available from the CMMS and the National Technical Information Service, Springfield, VA 22151, accession no. PB-179846.

7. Michael Pilot, "Health Manpower in 1980," *Occupational Outlook Quarterly*, Winter 1970, p. 3.

8. Harry I. Greenfield and Carol A. Brown, *Allied Health Manpower* (New York: Columbia University Press, 1969), p. 100.

9. Martha D. Ballenger and E. Harvey Estes, Jr., "Licensure or Responsible Delegation?" *New England Journal of Medicine*, Vol. 284, No. 6 (February 11, 1971), pp. 330-331.

10. Horowitz and Goldstein, *Hiring Standards for Paramedical Manpower*, pp. x-xi.

CHAPTER 3

1. Harold M. Goldstein and Morris A. Horowitz, *Restructuring Paramedical Occupations: Final Report* (Boston: Northeastern University, 1972, under a contract with the U.S. Department of Labor, Manpower Administration). The study is available from the National Technical Information Service, Springfield, VA 22151, accession nos. PB-211113 (vol. 1), PB-211114 (vol. 2—appendix C, Definition of Tasks and Functions; appendix D, Phase II tables, Analyzing the Functions Performed by Paramedical Personnel).

CHAPTER 6

1. Complete statistical data appear in Harold M. Goldstein and Morris A. Horowitz, *Utilization of Health Personnel: A Five Hospital Study*, Vol. 2 (appendix), a Report to the U.S. Department of Labor, Employment and Training Administration, March 1978, available from Government Printing Office, Washington, D.C. — National Technical Information Service.

2. *Ibid.*, tables A10-A12, pp. A99-A111.

3. *Ibid.*, tables A13-A15, pp. A112-A126.

4. *Ibid.*, tables A16-A18, pp. A127-A141.

5. *Ibid.*, tables A19-A22, pp. A142-A170.

6. *Ibid.*, tables A23-A26, pp. A171-A174.

7. *Ibid.*, tables A27-A29, pp. A175-A180.

8. U.S. Department of Labor, Bureau of Labor Statistics, *Occupational Outlook Handbook*, 1976-77 (Washington, D.C.: Government Printing Office, 1976), pp. 467-469.

9. Goldstein and Horowitz, *Utilization of Health Personnel: A Five Hospital Study*, Vol. II, tables A30-A32, pp. A181-A183.

10. *Ibid.*, table A33, pp.. A184-186.

11. *Ibid.*, table A34, pp A187.

12. *Ibid.*, tables A35-A38, pp. A188-A195.

CHAPTER 7

1. Harold M. Goldstein and Morris A. Horowitz, *Restructuring Paramedical Occupations,* a report to the U.S. Department of Labor, Manpower Administration, 1972, p. 46.

CHAPTER 8

1. A complete collection of functional questionnaires by the specific occupations analyzed in this study can be found in Vol. 2 of *Utilization of Health Personnel: A Five Hospital Study.*
2. For occupations and task definitions, see Goldstein and Horowitz, *Restructuring Paramedical Occupations,* Vol. 2, 1972.

CHAPTER 9

1. D.C. Feldman, "Organizational Socialization of Hospital Employees: A Comparative View of Occupational Groups," *Medical Care,* Vol. 15, No. 10 (1977), pp. 799-813.
2. *Ibid.,* p. 812.

Selected Bibliography

Alevizes, Gus; Walsh, Robert J.; and Aherne, Phil. *Socioeconomic Issues of Health*. Center for Health Services Research and Development. Chicago: American Medical Association, 1973.

American Hospital Association. *Hospitals,* Guide Issues. Chicago: American Hospital Association, annual, 1950-74.

_____ . *Survey of Hospital Charges as of January 1, 1974.* Chicago: American Hospital Association, 1974.

_____ . *Hospital Statistics.* Chicago: American Hospital Association, annual, 1972, 1973, 1974, 1977.

American Medical Association, Council on Medical Education. *Allied Medical Education Directory,* 1973. Chicago: American Medical Association, 1973.

_____ . *Medical Education in the United States 1972-1973.* Reprinted from *Journal of the American Medical Association,* 226,8 (November 19, 1973). Chicago: American Medical Association, 1973.

Ammer, Dean S. *Institutional Employment and Shortage of Paramedical Personnel: A Detailed Study of Staffing in Hospitals, Nursing Homes, and Various Institutions in the Greater Boston Area.* Grant from U.S. Public Health Service. Boston: Northeastern University, 1967.

Anderson, Odin W. *Health Care: Can There Be Equity? The United States, Sweden and England.* New York: John Wiley & Sons, 1972.

Baehr, George. "Some Popular Delusions about Health and Medical Care." *American Journal of Public Health* (March 1971), 582-586.

Baird, Charles W. "On Profits and Hospitals." *Journal of Economic Issues,* Vol. 5, No. 1 (March 1971), 57-67.

Ballenger, Martha D., and Estes, E. Harvey, Jr. "Licensure or

Responsible Delegation?" *New England Journal of Medicine,* Vol. 284, No. 6 (Feb. 11, 1971).

Berg, Robert L., M.D., ed. *Health Status Indexes.* Chicago: Hospital Research and Educational Trust, 1973.

Berki, Sylvester E. *Hospital Economics.* Lexington, Mass.: D. C. Heath and Co., Lexington Books, 1972.

Bicknell, William J., M.D., and Walsh, Diana C. "Certification-of-Need: The Massachusetts Experience." *New England Journal of Medicine,* Vol. 292, No. 20 (May 15, 1975), 1054-1061.

Burns, Eveline M. *Health Services for Tomorrow.* New York: Dunellen Publishing Co., 1973.

Committee for Economic Development. *Building a National Health Care System.* New York: Committee for Economic Development, April 1973.

Connecticut Institute for Health Manpower Resources, Inc. *Study of Educational Programs and Employment Opportunities in Health in Connecticut and the Northeast.* Hartford: Connecticut Institute for Health Manpower Resources, 1974.

Densen, Paul M. "Medical Schools and the Delivery of Medical Care to the Community." *New England Journal of Medicine* (May 20, 1971), 1156-1157.

DMI Health Manpower Information Exchange. *Documents Related to Health Manpower Planning: A Bibliography.* Preliminary Report. Washington, D.C.: Government Printing Office, 1974.

Doyle, Patrick J., M.D. *Save Your Health and Your Money.* Washington, D.C.: Acropolis Books, 1971.

Eilers, Robert D. "National Health Insurance: What Kind and How Much." *New England Journal of Medicine* (April 22, 1971), 881-887; (April 29, 1971), 945-955.

Executive Office of the President, Council on Wages and Price Stability. *The Problem of Rising Health Care Costs.* Staff Report. Washington, D.C.: Government Printing Office, 1976.

Fein, Rashi. "Can the 'Doctor Shortage' Be Solved?" *Hospital Practice* (April 1971), 73-101.

———. *The Doctor Shortage.* Washington, D.C.: Brookings Institution, 1967.

Fein, Rashi, and Weber, Gerald I. *Financing Medical Education.* A general report prepared for the Carnegie Commission on Higher Education and the Commonwealth Fund. New York: McGraw-Hill, 1971.

Feldman, D.C. "Organizational Socialization of Hospital Employees: A Comparative View of Occupational Groups." *Medical Care,* Vol. 15, No. 10 (1977).

Flexner, Abraham. *Medical Education in the United States and Canada.* Commissioned by the Carnegie Foundation for the Advancement of

Teaching, 1910. Reprint. Washington, D.C.: Science and Health Publications, 1960.

Franke, Walter and Sobel, Irvin. *The Shortage of Skilled and Technical Workers.* Lexington, Mass.: D.C. Heath and Co., Lexington Books, 1970.

Freeman, Howard E.; Levine, Sol; and Reeder, Leo G. *Handbook of Medical Sociology,* 2nd ed. Englewood, N.J.: Prentice Hall, 1972.

Fuchs, Victor R. *Who Shall Live?* New York: Basic Books, 1974.

Ginzberg, Eli, and the Conservation of Human Resources Staff, Columbia University. *Urban Health Services: The Case of New York.* New York: Columbia University Press, 1971.

Ginzberg, Eli, with Ostow, Miriam. *Men, Money and Medicine.* New York: Columbia University Press, 1969.

Goldstein, Harold M., and Horowitz, Morris A. *Employment and Utilization of Allied Medical Manpower in Hospitals.* Boston: Northeastern University, Department of Economics, Center for Medical Manpower Studies, 1976.

_____. *Entry-Level Health Occupations: Development and Future.* Baltimore: Johns Hopkins University Press, 1977.

_____. *Guide to Restructuring Medical Manpower Occupations in Hospitals.* Boston: Spaulding, 1975.

_____. *Health Manpower Employment.* A Report to the Office of Research and Development, Employment and Training Administration, U.S. Department of Labor, 1976.

_____. *Health Personnel: Meeting the Explosive Demand for Medical Care.* Germantown, Md.: Aspen Systems Corp., 1977.

_____. "Health Manpower — Shortage or Surplus?" *Journal of Allied Health,* 1974.

_____. *Paramedical Manpower: A Restructuring of Occupations.* Boston: Northeastern University, Department of Economics, 1972.

_____. *Research and Development in the Utilization of Medical Manpower.* Boston: Spaulding, 1974.

_____. *Restructuring Paramedical Occupations: Final Report,* 2 vols. U.S. Department of Labor, Manpower Administration, 1972.

_____. *Utilization of Health Personnel: A Five Hospital Study,* 2 vols. A report to the Office of Research and Development, Employment and Training Administration, U.S. Department of Labor, 1978.

Goldstein, Harold M.; Horowitz, Morris A.; Schachter, Gustav; Herrnstadt, Irwin L.; and Hankin, Robert A. *Health Manpower Literature,* Vol. 1, No. 1. Boston: Northeastern University, Department of Economics, Center for Medical Manpower Studies, 1977.

Goldstein, Harold M., and Schachter, Gustav. *Health Manpower: A United States Case Study in a Binational Perspective.* Access to Higher Education: Implication for International Manpower Planning, the Northeastern Center for International Higher Education Documentation, 1977.

Goldstein, Harold M.; Schachter, Gustav; and Hankin, Robert A. *Employment Prospects for Middle Echelon Health Care Administrators and Their Educational Implications,* A report for University of Massachusetts. Boston: Northeastern University, Department of Economics, Center for Medical Manpower Studies, 1976.

Gorman, Mike. "The Impact of National Health Insurance on the Development of Health Care." *American Journal of Public Health* (May 1971), 962-972.

Greenfield, Harry I. *Hospital Efficiency and Public Policy.* Center for Policy Research. New York: Praeger, 1973.

————, and Carol A. Brown. *Allied Health Manpower: Trends and Prospects.* New York: Columbia University Press, 1969.

Grossman, Michael. *The Demand for Health: A Theoretical and Empirical Investigation.* National Bureau of Economic Research, Occasional Paper 119. New York: Columbia University Press, 1972.

Horowitz, Morris A., and Goldstein, Harold M. *Hiring Standards for Paramedical Manpower.* A report to the Manpower Administration, U.S. Department of Labor. Boston: Northeastern University, 1968.

Keeler, Emmett B.; Newhouse, Joseph P.; and Phelps, Charles E. *Deductibles and the Demand for Medical Services: The Theory of the Consumer Facing a Variable Price Schedule under Uncertainty.* Santa Monica, Cal.: Rand Corporation, 1974.

Krizay, John, and Wilson, Andrew. *The Patient As Consumer.* A Twentieth Century Fund Report. Lexington, Mass.: D. C. Heath and Co., Lexington Books, 1974.

Lerner, Monroe, and Anderson, Odin W. *Health Progress in the United States: 1900-1960.* A Report of the Health Information Foundation. Chicago: University of Chicago Press, 1963.

Levey, Samuel, and Loomba, N. Paul. *Health Care Administration.* Philadelphia: J. B. Lippincott Co., 1973.

Luongo, Edward P., M.D. *American Medicine in Crisis.* New York: Philosophical Library, 1971.

Massachusetts, Commonwealth of, Department of Public Health. *Health Data Annual,* 1974, Vol. 1, No. 1. Boston: Massachusetts Department of Public Health, 1974.

————. Department of Public Health, Division of Medical Care, Bureau of Health Facilities. *Rules and Regulations for the Licensing of Long-Term Care Facilities.* Boston: Massachusetts Department of Public Health, 1971.

————, Executive Office for Administration and Finance. *Massachusetts Inventory of Published Statistical Series* Boston: Massachusetts Department of Public Health, 1970.

McCleery, Robert S., M.D. *One Life — One Physician.* Washington, D.C.: Public Affairs Press, 1971.

McCormick, James B., and Kopp, Joseph B. "Manpower Consideration/

Use of Technicians Frees Physicians." *Hospitals* (March 1971), 71-75.

McKinlay, John B., ed. *Economic Aspects of Health Care.* Milbank Memorial Fund. New York: Prodist, 1973.

Mendelson, Mary Adelaide. *Tender Loving Greed.* New York: Alfred A. Knopf, 1974.

Morreale, Joseph C., ed. *The U.S. Medical Care Industry: The Economist's Point of View.* Michigan Business Papers Number 60. Ann Arbor: University of Michigan, 1974.

Mueller, Marjorie Smith, and Gibson, Robert M. "National Health Expenditures, Fiscal Year 1975." *Social Security Bulletin 32, No. 2, 18.*

National Academy of Sciences, *Cost of Education in the Health Professions,* Pts. 1,2, and 3. Washington, D.C.: Government Printing Office, 1974.

National Commission on Accrediting. *Study of Accreditation of Selected Health Educational Programs.* Commission Report. Washington, D.C.: National Commission on Accrediting, 1972.

National Planning Association, Center for Health Policy Studies. *Chartbooks of Federal Health Spending.* Washington, D.C.: Government Printing Office, 1974.

Navarro, Vincente. "Health and Corporate Society." *Social Policy* (January/February 1975), 41.

Newhouse, Joseph P. *Forecasting Demand for Medical Care for the Purpose of Planning Health Services.* Santa Monica, Cal.: Rand Corporation, 1974.

Newhouse, Joseph P., and Phelps, Charles E. *On Having Your Cake and Eating It Too: Econometric Problems in Estimating the Demand for Health Services.* Santa Monica, Cal.: Rand Corporation, 1974.

Newhouse, Joseph P.; Phelps, Charles E.; and Schwartz, William B. "Policy Options and the Impact of National Health Insurance." *New England Journal of Medicine* (June 13, 1974), 1345-1359.

Organization for Economic and Community Development. *New Directions in Education for Changing Health Systems.* Paris: Organization for Economic and Community Development, 1975.

Penchansky, Roy, ed. *Health Services Administration.* Cambridge, Mass.: Harvard University Press, 1968.

Perlman, Mark, ed. *The Economics of Health and Medical Care.* New York: John Wiley & Sons, 1974.

Pharmaceutical Manufacturers Association. *Fact Book.* Washington, D.C.: Pharmaceutical Manufacturers Association, 1972.

Phelps, Charles E. *Demand for Health Insurance: A Theoretical and Empirical Investigation.* Santa Monica, Cal.: Rand Corporation, 1973.

Phelps, Charles E., and Newhouse, Joseph P. *Coinsurance and the Demand for Medical Services.* Santa Monica, Cal.: Rand Corporation, 1974.

Pratt, Lois. "The Relationship of Socio-Economic Status to

Health." *American Journal of Public Health* (February 1971), 281-292.

Rice, Dorothy P., and McGee, Mary F. "Projections of National Health Expenditures, 1975 and 1980." *Research and Statistics,* Note No. 18 (October 30, 1970). Washington, D.C.: Government Printing Office, 1970.

Roemer, Milton I., and Friedman, Jay W. *Doctors in Hospitals.* Baltimore: John Hopkins University Press, 1971.

Rosenberg, William E. "Who's Out of Date?" *New England Journal of Medicine* (April 15, 1971), 850-851.

Rutstein, David D., M.D. *The Coming Revolution in Medicine.* Cambridge, Mass.: MIT Press, 1974.

––––––. *Blueprint for Medical Care.* Cambridge, Mass.: MIT Press, 1974.

Schechter, Daniel S. *Agenda for Continuing Education.* Chicago: Hospital Research and Educational Trust, 1974.

Scott, W. Richard, and Volkart, Edmund H., eds. *Medical Care Readings in the Sociology of Medical Institutions.* New York: John Wiley & Sons, 1966.

Sidenstricker, Edgar. *The Challenge of Facts: Selected Public Health Papers,* edited by Richard V. Kasius. Milbank Memorial Fund. New York: Prodist, 1974.

Sigerist, Henry E. *On the Sociology of Medicine,* edited by Milton I. Roemer, M.D. New York: MD Publications, 1960.

Skolik, Alfred M., and Dales, Sophie R. "Social Welfare Expenditures, 1968-1969." *Social Security Bulletin 32* (December 1969), 12.

Somers, Herman M., and Somers, Anne R. *Medicare and the Hospitals.* Washington, D.C.: Brookings Institution, 1967.

Sorkin, Alan L. *Health Economics.* Lexington, Mass.: D. C. Heath and Co., Lexington Books, 1975.

Steward, Charles T., Jr. "Allocations of Resources to Health." *Journal of Human Resources* (Winter 1971), 103-123.

Stuart, Craig, and Barrett, H. Lee, Jr. "Medicaid and Boston's Neighborhood Health Centers: Integrating Two Concepts of Health Care." Unpublished paper submitted to Professor Lloyd L. Weinre for Seminar on Institutional Change in Urban American, Harvard University, April 1972.

Tribble, William D. *Doctor Draft Justified.* San Antonio, Texas: National Biomedical Laboratories, 1968.

United Nations Statistical Office. *Statistical Yearbook.* New York: United Nations, annual, 1972, 1974.

U.S. Department of Commerce. *Business Statistics,* 1973. Washington, D.C.: Government Printing Office, 1973.

––––––. *Survey of Current Business,* 54, 4. Washington, D.C.: Government Printing Office, 1974.

––––––. Bureau of the Census. *Census of Population: 1970.* Vol. 1,

PC(1)-D1, United States Summary, Detailed Characteristics. Washington, D.C.: Government Printing Office, 1970.

_____. *Statistical Abstract of the United States,* 1974. Washington, D.C.: Government Printing Office, 1973 and 1974.

U.S. Department of Health, Education, and Welfare, National Center for Health Statistics. *Characteristics of Residents in Nursing and Personal Care Homes, United States — June-August 1969.* Vital and Health Statistics, Series 12, No. 19. Washington, D.C.: Government Printing Office, 1973.

_____. *Charges for Care in Nursing Homes: United States — August-September 1968.* Vital and Health Statistics, Series 12, No. 14. Washington, D.C.: Government Printing Office, 1972.

_____. *Employees in Nursing Homes: United States — April-September 1968.* Vital and Health Statistics, Series 12, No. 15. Washington, D.C.: Government Printing Office, 1972.

_____. *Health Manpower Sources Book 21.* Washington, D.C.: Government Printing Office, 1970.

_____. *Health Resources Statistics.* Washington, D.C.: Government Printing Office, annual 1969, 1972, 1973, 1974.

_____. "1973-74 Nursing Home Survey: Provisional Data." Monthly Vital Statistics Report, HRA 75-1120. Washington, D.C.: Government Printing Office, 1974.

_____. *Selected Characteristics of Nursing Homes for the Aged and Chronically Ill: United States — June-August 1969.* Vital and Health Statistics, Series 12, No. 23. Washington, D.C.: Government Printing Office, 1974.

_____. *Utilization of Institutions for the Aged and Chronically Ill: United States — April-June 1963.* Vital and Health Statistics, Series 12, No. 4. Washington, D.C.: Government Printing Office, 1966.

U.S. Department of Health, Education, and Welfare, Social Security Administration. *Calendar 1972 Highlights.* By Barbara S. Cooper, Nancy L. Worthington, and Paula Piro. Washington, D.C.: Government Printing Office, 1974.

_____. *Compendium of National Health Expenditure Data.* By Barbara S. Cooper, Nancy Worthington, and Mary McGee. Washington, D.C.: Government Printing Office, 1972.

_____. *Health Insurance Statistics,* 1968-72. Washington, D.C.: Government Printing Office, annual.

_____. *Research and Statistics,* Note No. 3, 1973. Washington, D.C.: Government Printing Office, 1973.

_____. *Social Security Bulletin,* December 1972. Washington, D.C.: Government Printing Office, 1972.

U.S. Department of Labor and U.S. Department of Health, Education, and Welfare. *Manpower Report of the President,* 1974. Washington, D.C.: Government Printing Office, 1974.

U.S. Department of Labor, Bureau of Labor Statistics. *Annual Earnings and Employment Patterns of Private Nonagricultural Employees, 1965.* Bulletin 1675. Washington, D.C.: Government Printing Office, 1971.

_____ . *Consumer Price Index for Selected Items and Groups, Monthly and Annual Averages.* Washington, D.C.: Government Printing Office, annual, 1950-72.

_____ . *Employment and Earnings.* Washington, D.C.: Government Printing Office, monthly 1950-73.

_____ . "Employment in the Medical and Other Health Services." Based on unpublished data from U.S. Department of Commerce. *Statistical Abstract of the United States* 1973, Table No. 107.

_____ . *Industry and Wage Survey, Hospitals, March 1969.* Bulletin 1688. Washington, D.C.: Government Printing Office: 1971.

_____ . *Occupational Outlook Handbook,* 1976-77. Washington, D.C.: Government Printing Office, 1976.

_____ . *Occupational Outlook Quarterly,* Vol. 14, No. 4. Washington, D.C.: Government Printing Office, 1970.

_____ . *Tomorrow's Manpower Needs,* Vol. 4, rev. Washington, D.C.: Government Printing Office, 1971.

University of Michigan School of Public Health. *The Report of the Commission on Education for Health Administration,* Vol. 1 ("Kellogg Report"). Ann Arbor, Mich.: Health Administration Press, 1975.

Vahovich, Steve G., ed. *Profile of Medical Practice, 1973.* Chicago: Center for Health Services Research and Development, American Medical Association, 1973.

Ward, Richard A. *The Economics of Health Resources.* Reading, Mass.: Addison-Wesley, 1975.

Wilson, Florence A., and Newhauser, Duncan. *Health Services in the United States.* Cambridge, Mass.: Ballenger, 1974.

Yett, Donald E. *An Economic Analysis of the Nurse Shortage.* Lexington, Mass.: D. C. Heath and Co., Lexington Books, 1975.

Index